Fat Planet

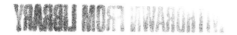

School for Advanced Research
Advanced Seminar Series
Michael F. Brown
General Editor

Since 1970 the School for Advanced Research
(formerly the School of American Research)
and SAR Press have published over one hundred
volumes in the Advanced Seminar Series. These
volumes arise from seminars held on SAR's
Santa Fe campus that bring together small
groups of experts to explore a single issue.
Participants assess recent innovations in theory
and methods, appraise ongoing research, and
share data relevant to problems of significance
in anthropology and related disciplines. The
resulting volumes reflect SAR's commitment to
the development of new ideas and to scholarship
of the highest caliber. The complete Advanced
Seminar Series can be found at www.sarweb.org.

Fat Planet

OBESITY, CULTURE, AND
SYMBOLIC BODY CAPITAL

Edited by Eileen P. Anderson-Fye and Alexandra Brewis

SCHOOL FOR ADVANCED RESEARCH PRESS • SANTA FE

UNIVERSITY OF NEW MEXICO PRESS • ALBUQUERQUE

Library of Congress Cataloging-in-Publication Data

Names: Anderson-Fye, Eileen P., editor. | Brewis, Alexandra A., 1965– editor.
Title: Fat planet : obesity, culture, and symbolic body capital / edited by Eileen P. Anderson-Fye
and Alexandra Brewis.
Description: Santa Fe : School for Advanced Research Press ; Albuquerque : University of New
Mexico Press, 2017. | Series: School for Advanced Research Advanced Seminar Series | Includes
bibliographical references and index.
Identifiers: LCCN 2016021326 (print) | LCCN 2016059338 (ebook) | ISBN 9780826358004
(paperback) | ISBN 9780826358011 (electronic)
Subjects: LCSH: Obesity—Social aspects. | Medical anthropology. | BISAC: SOCIAL SCIENCE /
Anthropology / Cultural. | SOCIAL SCIENCE / Sociology / General.
Classification: LCC RC628.F332 2017 (print) | LCC RC628 (ebook) | DDC 362.1963/98—dc23
LC record available at https://lccn.loc.gov/2016021326

Cover photo: *Fat embolism* by Yale Rosen licensed
under CC by 2.0

Composed in Minion Pro and Gill Sans

This book is the outcome of a long process, made possible through multiple organizations. First, Arizona State University and Case Western Reserve University supported the early seeds of this collaboration. The National Science Foundation Cultural Anthropology Program supported exploratory research on the ethnography of comparative fat stigma born of conversations among the coeditors. Program officers Deborah Winslow and Jeffrey Mantz have been remarkable in their diligence and feedback, making the results better. Chapter 3 by Anderson-Fye et al. is based upon work supported by the National Science Foundation under Grant Number BCS-1244944. Any opinions, findings, and conclusions or recommendations expressed in this material are those of the authors and do not necessarily reflect the views of the National Science Foundation.

This volume was brought to fruition through the generous support and hospitality of the School for Advanced Research (SAR). In March 2014, nine of us gathered together for a week in frigid but beautiful Santa Fe, being fully cared for by the extraordinary team at the SAR seminar house. The SAR experience allowed our collective ideas to take hold and grow, and it is why this book exists. We met our goal that week—to bring together thinkers who would engage different levels of analysis, theoretical perspectives, and methodologies in exploration of issues related to the body norms that relate to obesity in multiple regions of the world. In particular, we sought to advance our understanding of the role of obesity as a symbolic and material entity, along with its constantly changing meanings and outcomes. Through the conversations within the advanced seminar, we were also able to push forward a further and perhaps more important agenda—to add the anthropology of obesity to a more central position within the often frenzied global obesity discourse. The editors could not have asked for a more collegial and productive group. We also thank the staff at SAR for continuing to support and encourage our collective efforts long after we left the seminar house. In particular, former program officer Nicole L. Taylor was a voice of both substantive and process wisdom. SAR is a unique and important institution advancing social science in a quiet but extraordinarily powerful way—by fostering good ideas to percolate, interlocute, and grow so they can be better.

The individual authors in this volume appreciate the generous funding of their work from several sources. In particular, the data presented in chapter 5 were supported by a National Science Foundation Doctoral Dissertation Research Improvement Grant (BCS-0922436) awarded to Eileen P. Anderson-Fye and Stephanie M. McClure and the Ford and Spencer Foundations, which also supported McClure's larger dissertation project. Nicole L. Taylor's work in chapter 6 was funded in part by a grant from the Department of Anthropology at the University of Arizona and a dissertation fellowship from the American Association of University Women. Chapter 7 by Anne E. Becker included data from a study supported by the National Institutes of Health (K23 MH068575). The larger project from which chapter 8 is drawn was also supported by a National Science Foundation Doctoral Dissertation Research Improvement Grant (BCS-0851478) awarded to Ivy L. Pike and Sarah Trainer.

We also are extremely grateful for the editorial work of the Global Fat Stigma team at Case Western Reserve University, and of Erika Jerme, whose work was made possible through the Mayo Clinic–ASU Obesity Solutions initiative and funding provided by the Virginia G. Piper Charitable Trust.

Making Sense of the New Global Body Norms

ALEXANDRA BREWIS

One of the most profound biological changes for the human species has been the consistent rise in average body mass over the last several decades. In 2015, the World Health Organization reported that some two billion adults were overweight or obese.[1] In all but the poorest nations in sub-Saharan Africa, technically overweight and obese bodies are becoming the new biological norm (Ng et al. 2014). From Fiji to Jamaica, and the United Arab Emirates to the United States, the average adult's body mass index (BMI) is now well into the overweight range. In eight countries—four in the central Pacific and four in the Persian Gulf and North Africa—more than 75 percent of the adult population is overweight or obese. Current accelerating trends in childhood overweight, and the increasing recognition that no one has yet devised any strategy that can reverse obesity at the national level, suggest we all will live in an even fatter planet in the decades ahead (Roberto 2015).

Historically, only the very wealthiest and most powerful had sufficient excess of food and leisure to become overweight or obese. But in recent decades, particularly since World War II, our shrinking world has led to rapidly expanding bodies. Major processes of modernization—including economic growth, market integration, trade liberalization, technological advancement, mechanization, and urbanization—have made high-calorie, high-fat foods cheaper and more accessible (Popkin, Adair, and Ng 2012). These *globalizing* processes have also changed how we organize our work, transport, and leisure time, much of it toward more sitting and less physical activity. As more households engage with the global market economy, take cash employment, and become new global consumers, they tend to become increasingly sedentary and eat more processed foods—and gain additional weight as a result. This historical trend of collective weight gain started sooner and developed more slowly in the wealthiest nations. But now that it has begun to reach into middle- and even lower-income nations, the speed at which these populations are gaining weight is accelerating as national wealth grows (Hruschka and Brewis 2012).

More recently, however, wealthier nations have followed a different trajectory: as overall wealth and wealth disparities increase, obesity risk has slid down the socioeconomic ladder. We now observe clustering of obesity (and related chronic diseases, such as diabetes) with other compounding markers of social or economic marginalization in wealthier nations such as Australia, the United Kingdom, and the United States. In neighborhoods where incomes are lower, affordable healthy food choices are fewer, exercise opportunities are more limited, and health care is less accessible (e.g., El-Sayed, Scarborough, and Galea 2012). Middle-income nations, such as India and China, appear to be experiencing the beginnings of this same reversal, suggesting that in such countries obesity also will become tied to need, poverty, and vulnerability rather than plenty, wealth, and security (Dinsa et al. 2012).

Concerned by the association between obesity and expensive, deadly chronic diseases such as diabetes and cardiovascular disease, affluent nations of the global north have been fighting a desperate public health and medical "war on obesity" for several decades. These campaigns are now spreading throughout the developing world. But often this massive effort to tackle the "obesity epidemic" looks and feels more like a campaign against fat people themselves (Hansen 2014). At the same time, the social meaning of obese bodies also appears to be shifting rapidly across the world. In a key study based on global data we collected in 2010, we identified fat bodies emerging as a sudden and new, globally shared, moral preoccupation across a wide array of societies. From Mexico and American Samoa to the United States and New Zealand, people expressed negative, judgmental ideas about obese bodies, seemingly as a core cultural norm (Brewis et al. 2011). This global trend toward fat stigma has happened quickly—so quickly that even those of us conducting field research around body norms almost missed it. Over the preceding decades, several of us have conducted detailed ethnographic studies in places where large and curvy bodies were generally viewed in positive terms (Anne E. Becker in Fiji [1995, 2004], Alexandra A. Brewis in Samoa [1998, 2000], Eileen P. Anderson-Fye in Belize [2004]); many other examples also exist in the ethnographic record. These bodies were seen as representing power, beauty, sexual appeal, wealth, social connection, and caring. The sudden, generally unanticipated switch to globalized fat stigma has happened with exceptional speed, most of it seemingly within the decade. And this shift is happening even as physically obese bodies become more common.

We term these negative attitudes *fat stigma*. We use the word *fat* as a social category or social fact that is deployed subjectively as a descriptor of specific physical bodies. This is in contrast to our utilization of *obesity*, a term that refers to medicalized perspectives on and definitions of large body size. Obesity usually relies on body mass indices and similar standardized measures (see Brewis 2011 for an extended discussion).

The concept of stigma has a long history in social science (beginning with and often circling back to Erving Goffman), and the construct often focuses on the process of an arbitrary characteristic of the individual becoming both socially undesirable and morally discredited. In this manner, the stigma of "being fat" is one of the most significant of modern life, laden with derogatory meaning; the phrase evokes such descriptors as lazy, dirty, unsexy, and unlovable. Ethnographic studies in wealthier Western nations have detailed the devastating emotional suffering such attitudes cause for people labeled as "too fat." Meera and Riccardi (2008) provide particularly compelling accounts of the anguish felt in sharing the stories of bariatric patients preparing for surgery. Fat stigma seems especially prone to internalization as self-blame. And this sense of guilt is tied tightly to the core expressed belief (such as in anti-obesity campaigns or even clinical practice) that obesity is first and best modified by individual efforts. As a result, individual culpability is easily placed by everyone—including those with large bodies themselves—onto people socially stained as "being too fat."

The recent anti-obesity campaigns emerging around the globe tend to describe fat as dangerous and in turn seem to advance the spread of fat stigma (Brewis and Wutich 2014; Campos et al. 2006). In addition, the globalization of social media appears to be part of the trend and helps explain *how* people are exposed to new norms. Nevertheless, these elements alone do not explain fully *why* people would adopt these new body norms with such enthusiasm. As part of our search for an answer, Eileen Anderson-Fye and I organized a School for Advanced Research (SAR) seminar in March 2014. The contributors to this volume participated in that weeklong collaborative effort in Santa Fe to explore this increasingly timely and relevant question. The week's conversations featured a range of perspectives from the fields of anthropology, sociology, psychology, and psychiatry. That transdisciplinarity proved invaluable to developing a more comprehensive and broad theorization of the fat body as a social and economic agent in the modern world.

During the seminar, we identified a number of transecting themes and issues. First, we used the term *fat stigma* to grapple with these changing norms around large bodies and the increasingly negative and judgmental social reaction to them. Yet traditional approaches to stigma as a construct proved weak theoretical tools for understanding the cross-cultural and temporal complexity of new body norms around fat. The concept of stigma has a long and fairly conventional history in sociology and psychology. Much of the theory building involved was tied to understanding the treatment of people with mental illness and certain infectious diseases such as HIV/AIDS. In these realms, stigma is conceptualized as structurally created, such as through institutional messaging and rituals (e.g., advertising or organizational patterns in hospital routines). This conceptualization is sometimes explained as "stigma power": the capacity to keep some people down or out for the benefit of others, legitimizing exclusions and discriminations and reinforcing advantaged positions within the social hierarchy (Parker and Aggleton 2003).

There are many examples of how this conventional approach applies adequately in the domain of fat stigma in general, including a stated disdain by many in the medical professions for treating "noncompliant" patients with high body weight, the failure to enact laws against discrimination on the basis of weight despite repeatedly documented exclusions, and disparities in education and employment opportunities between those with larger versus smaller bodies. Stigma is also traditionally theorized as emerging interpersonally, in the day-to-day interactions people have with friends, families, and strangers; the frequency of stares and rude comments people struggling with high weights receive clearly illustrates the interpersonal nature of fat stigma.

Yet to understand fully *why* fat stigma is gaining such traction and to articulate how it is shaping people's lives across the globe, we have to think between and beyond such analytic lenses and explore the meanings of fat as they vary across and interact among a vast array of contexts. We must include in our analysis such factors as modern marriage and economic markets at both the local and global scales, the multiple other vulnerabilities or points of difference (e.g., ethnicity) that layer onto or connect with embodied identities, and the prioritization (or not) of fat-avoidant body projects in the face of the many other constraints and concerns people face every day.

Accordingly, for the new theory building we are doing here, we decided to use *fat stigma* as a general term rather than be constrained by the more technically concise definitions usually employed in existing disciplinary stigma research. This decision was purposeful and important. Throughout the text, you will see people use terms such as *fat stigma, obesity stigma, thin body ideals*, or *body norms* to reflect the multitude of ways that the authors draw on diverse understandings of fat stigma and body norms as they frame their work.

Other important consistencies emerged during our SAR conversations with regard to how we came to understand the ways that fat becomes socially excluded. For example, we agreed that the moral meanings surrounding fat stigma allow us to identify and isolate the relevant social norms. We also found that people across the globe seem almost universally aware that fat is "bad" and exhibit surprising convergence in their body norms. By *body norms*, we mean what people generally, collectively agree is normal, acceptable, or desirable. Thus fat stigmas reflect and reinforce "what matters most" in social terms (Yang et al. 2014) to people, such as a marriageable, hirable body—that is, one that possesses high symbolic capital convertible into what people want or need. We observed that the attention to avoiding fat stigma is constant and obvious in the wide array of contexts—from Fijian villages to American school yards—explored in this volume, and that it isn't just people at high weights who are concerned about and affected by this stigma.

The massive amount of time and energy that millions devote to weight loss perhaps reflects not so much an urge for health as avoidance of the cost of being socially discredited as "too fat" or achievement of the relative social advantages of "thin enough." Thus fear of fat stigma seems to be a major motivator for people to work very hard to try to align with body norms as closely as they can.

Consideration of what the *fat* body in particular means in cultural, social, moral, and practical terms has not been the focus of stigma research to date. In addition, anthropological investigations of body norms more generally have little discussed notions of stigma. Rather, prior analyses concentrated on what ethnographic fieldwork until recently yielded—growing concerns with thinness. Much of the theorizing about body norms in anthropology and related fields has centered on these concerns, but we find it limiting to theorize fat stigma as being merely the flip side of thin idealism. The studies presented are highly influenced by, but step well away from, the cross-cultural literature on body norms (such as represented in the prior work of Anderson-Fye and Becker in this volume), which has emphasized growing slim idealism across the globe over the last generation. We worked hard to not be bound by this literature and found at the end of the seminar and our collective discussions that we need to rethink "being fat" in cultural terms as much more and different than "not being thin." This perspective has helped us identify some new and important theoretical points—perhaps most especially the idea that people can hold more than one and even competing body norms at the same time. Similarly, we found that the concept of fat stigma also needs to better accommodate the idea that stigmas are rarely singular: they tend to intersect or layer with multiple structural vulnerabilities such as poverty, sexism, racism, and so on.

To begin to address directly the question of why fat stigma is spreading so fast, we focused on the role of local and global economic change. In particular, we looked at individual concerns regarding upward mobility as a starting point to begin to unpack the *why*. As the seminar proceeded, our discussions quickly widened to incorporate ideas of power in relation to the meaning of large bodies. Specifically, we sought to deepen our understanding of the meanings and norms of the body as a potential tool for upward mobility or socioeconomic advantage—that is, the application of symbolic body capital. Conversely, some bodies in some contexts can create barriers to advancement, or even reverse existing opportunities.

If over time we became more slippery in our deployment of the term *fat stigma* to allow greater theoretical experimentation, we also became much more tightly focused in how we discussed and operationalized this economic and advancement context. Elizabeth Sweet (2011) detailed a model of the symbolic capital of consumption (material display of social status and its social constraint) as existing at the intersection of macro- and micropolitical economic change and potentially stress-inducing cultural norms. Her model provides a useful addendum to this working theory. Sweet's framework does not consider the notions of symbolic capital specifically in the context of larger versus smaller bodies, but does provide a conceptual, and potentially testable, link between the issues of large body size, body-image change (and possible concomitant resistance), and economic changes at the macro and micro level. For example, as larger bodies become the norm, the *symbolic capital* model suggests two simultaneous reactions will follow: one against what is a likely erosion of the large body as an acceptable marker of social capital or another in favor of smaller bodies as a new one. This construct was key to how we bridged our individual work into a comparative, collaborative effort to understand fat stigma that connects our work across very diverse places and involves very different levels and modes of analysis.

We also specified that by *upward mobility*, we mean the drive to improve one's social status, economic status, or both. In sociological terms, upward mobility can engage various forms of *capital* or resources—economic, cultural, human, social, physical, and symbolic. We draw on the ideas of Pierre Bourdieu (1984) with regard to the non-economic social assets driving upward mobility. In particular, we focus on the role of goods (which could include body size) that are rare and worthy of being acquired to mark status. Thus, in a time of scarcity, a fat body that consumes resources with relatively low exertion would be unusual and desirable. In a contemporary world with increasing urbanization and abundant and cheap lower-quality foods (in relation to health outcomes), a slender body can be seen as one that can afford fresh foods and the leisure pursuit of exercise. Moreover, especially for bodies gendered masculine, the global proliferation of a muscular body ideal includes assumptions of enough time and "work" on the body to achieve the ideal (e.g., Pope, Phillips, and Olivardia 2000). Increasingly, educational achievement is a key part of opportunity for upward mobility throughout the world. If people cannot easily access this pathway (for reasons such as limited finances), the role of symbolic capital as a means of upward mobility should be even more important to them.

So this book explores new ground to understand the ways increasingly fatter bodies are morally understood and used and abused in our increasingly complex globalized, capitalized, liberalized, and materialized world. As we show, evolving and seemingly expanding cultural norms about what bigger bodies mean, and related ideas of blame, are set within multiple intersecting global processes that play out locally: the democratization of education; the push to urban centers or transnational migrations to succeed in the cash economy; the spread of Internet access and, with it, engagement in new forms of social influence and types of dating markets; and the increasing entrenchment of inequality within nations reinforced through a dizzying array of institutional structures.

But this volume is also designed to help reboot our thinking around how anthropologists are reacting to and commenting on the growing global "obesity epidemic." Most of the existing anthropological literature has focused on the impact of both larger bodies and social reactions to those bodies in the United States and other advanced anglophone economies. This work fails to acknowledge that the "fattest" nations are actually mostly in the rest of the world. To better understand what it means to be a fatter *planet*, we actually need to include the entire globe within our broad theorization. This approach may seem obvious, but it is not how the field has generally moved—perhaps in part driven by a conventional but incorrect wisdom that the West is where most of the problematic body fat is concentrated.

Moreover, a concerning polemic has emerged around how we talk about fat in academic circles. Much of the anthropological, sociological, and fat studies scholarship pushes against the medical and public health notion of fat as unhealthy and instead rails against the proposition that this "obesity epidemic" will doom us all. We need to find new ways to speak to both of these concerns in constructive, meaningful ways. We need the frameworks that embrace this social critique of the fat body as a damaging social fact without denying that—however poorly or even destructively they may be expressed in social terms—the biological and medical observations about the health risks of excess weight also are valid and need to be addressed (Trainer et al. 2015b). Certainly, it is the only way our efforts as social scientists will spur concrete interventions for people and societies around the world. This book is our effort to forge that more neutral and inclusive theoretical space, to bridge that chasm between fat as a biological and social fact and to do what is needed to more deeply engage in the complexities of what is *really* going on with fat on our planet.

STRUCTURE OF THE BOOK

This chapter describes the origins of this book, specifically the core questions driving our exploration of the rapid expansion and embrace of these new body norms. The chapters that follow ask: How is the meaning of fat transforming globally and how does this transformation relate to other intersecting processes that also play out locally and globally—including globalization, socioeconomic development, and shifting economic opportunities? Specifically, how do new body norms shape opportunities for upward mobility or otherwise shape and reshape power relations? The authors of this volume purposefully shift among diverse levels of analysis and employ different theories to unpack the intersections of fatter (and thinner) bodies, the symbolic (and other) body capital they contain, and their means of upward mobility.

Daniel J. Hruschka provides a broad context for the chapters that follow by presenting a cross-national analysis that clarifies how changing body mass and wealth are related at the population level. His integrative approach, drawing on training at the intersection of mathematics, human biology, and medical anthropology, explicitly tests basic social and evolutionary theories against one another to expose the underlying drivers of body-wealth associations. His analysis begins with historical observations of a general pattern of positive relationships between increasing wealth and increasing body size, most visible at the national level. Since the 1980s, however, we have begun to observe inversions of this association, particularly in developed nations. Greater wealth is becoming associated with lower body mass, whereas poverty is increasingly linked to obesity risk. Hruschka analyzes large, cross-national data sets to test two competing theories. The first involves the directional relationship between upward mobility and body size—that income and wealth better allow women to change their behavior to meet new norms. The second is that women's greater capacity to meet the new slim body norms leads to increased wealth. He suggests a specific and critical mechanism that underlies the broad observed population-level patterns: marriage markets increasingly act to sort thinner women into higher-income households. He also notes the importance of interpreting such broad, population-level findings within the particularities and constraints of local dating and marriage markets.

Chapter 2 clarifies and expands upon these questions. Anthropologist Alexander Edmonds and sociologist Ashley Mears use intersecting social analyses to explicate the idea of symbolic body capital more fully as it applies locally and globally. Their work focuses specifically on young women with beauty to "sell." The two combine insights from their own previous works (e.g., Edmonds 2010) with Bourdieu's theories to show the ways young people use the body while they navigate the complexities of capitalism through the worth assigned to aesthetic attractiveness. Fat is one key, globalizing component of beauty in modern markets (marital, labor, or otherwise), although their analysis also considers others. They note that we always need to examine who owns the capital that slim beauty creates. In the case of women in VIP lounges, for example, the benefits of extensive and often unhealthy efforts to increase "girl capital" do not always accrue to the girls themselves. Thus the markets that potentially benefit women also create vulnerabilities by virtue of the lengths to which people go to gain aesthetic power, as well as the possibility that such power will be quickly appropriated by others.

In chapter 3, psychological and medical anthropologist Eileen P. Anderson-Fye and colleagues use a cross-cultural and comparative framework to present a thematic analysis of ethnographic data from three countries. This research helps illuminate the ways young adults experience and apply body norms—and in turn how those local ideas affect upward mobility. By applying extensive qualitative and ethnographic approaches to Belize, Jamaica, and Nepal, they found data that underscore the fluid, and sometimes contradictory, nature of fat stigma. That is, the nature and intensity of fat stigma vary tremendously even within the same community or family, and certainly between developing and fully rural areas. This chapter highlights the importance of recognizing that myriad factors affect and shape fat stigma; scholars and policy makers both must resist the temptation to oversimplify explanations and interventions. Fat stigma differentially affects and is leveraged by people within communities—males or females, lower or higher incomes, college educated or not. What size and shape is deemed "too fat" in one context of people's everyday lives might be acceptable or even appealing in another. Even as we reach for middle-range or higher theory to explain globalizing fat stigma, elemental understandings of how people manage these meanings as they go through their daily lives, connect to others, and reach for their own goals remain central. Reactions to our own and others' fat are always personal and local. The findings from Nepal in particular provide a valuable balance to the broader theory Hruschka presents in chapter 1: the results there illustrate that people can be extremely concerned about weight with regard to their own prospects yet disconnect its importance from concerns about marriage markets.

In chapter 4, feminist sociologist Monica J. Casper explores the ways that women's vulnerabilities are shaped and how power is reinforced through social and political reactions to fat. She uses her work on the *invisibility* of infant mortality as a health crisis in the United States to underscore the *hypervisibility* of obesity. Casper also shows how the two "crises" intersect at the site of (overweight, minority) women's wombs. She also demonstrates how notions of blame attached to obesity are embedded in the politics of disadvantage in the United States, producing and masking the lack of women's autonomy, especially for those already disadvantaged by poverty, race, or immigrant status. The hypervisibility of fat in public discussion of health and health disparities leads to constant surveillance and discrimination. The biopolitical gaze is focused on women's *weight*, and especially expectant mothers' weight, as the problem that must be solved. Instead, Casper posits, attention should be paid to the unjust structural factors that create the risk of women's weight gain to begin with.

Tackling the oft-cited countercase in the body-image literature of African American women's bodies, cultural and medical anthropologist Stephanie M.

McClure discusses her ethnographic study in the American Midwest in chapter 5. Body-image literature tends to pose African American women's cultural body norms as an exception, given their low rates of reported body dissatisfaction compared to other groups. In their historically placed position on the *margins* of broader body markets, McClure explains, young African American women's understandings of symbolic body capital are not as much racialized as situational. The lived experience of bodies, and the power they can have, centers on navigating being on the margins and being "not the norm." Her work challenges assumptions about how African American girls navigate weight and suggests struggles within that process. Her work explores how these young women understand and react to the male gaze; it also highlights the need to understand the diffuse nature of their body ideals—focused on general presentation rather than the specifics of size or shape. McClure's analysis also offers ties to some of the key themes from Casper's analysis of marginalized and racialized obese bodies; by including ethnographic observations from a personal and lived rather than a biopolitical, analytic lens, McClure also illustrates ways that these women manage to express some control and agency as they navigate the ambiguities of that marginalization and visibility of their bodies, fat and otherwise.

In chapter 6, linguistic anthropologist Nicole L. Taylor also focuses on a single ethnographic case to address body norms in American youth. Her analysis attends to the gendered language of fat, especially how it is employed to create and reinforce important social hierarchies. Like McClure, Taylor shows how youth "try on" or negotiate different body-related identities as they move among different social cliques within a high school in the Southwest. She explains how girls, again, are especially vulnerable to discipline (in both the literal and Foucaultian sense) when they fail to meet presentation norms. Many of their accounts involved experiences within female peer groups, meaning the female gaze was at least as important as a male one. Girls who could construct themselves as thin (the imagined body) rose in the social hierarchy, regardless of exact level of thinness (the material body). Their opportunities for upward mobility—as well as for avoidance of exclusion or other social costs—rests at the intersection of acceptable physical bodies and ways they shape attendant moral meanings to achieve social advantage.

In chapter 7, medical anthropologist and psychiatrist Anne E. Becker examines ways that the body's influence on symbolic capital is revealed at the family and community level. Becker has conducted ethnographic research in Sigatoka, Fiji, since the 1980s. Her more recent work has provided the most detailed ethnographic analyses of how body image has changed amid multiple global changes (migration, urbanization, economic development, and assimilation) over the last several decades and considers how these intersecting processes relate to young women's aspirations for upward mobility. Here Becker explains how the meanings and moral attributions of ambition, and the uncontrolled eating that might derail it, are configured as a social (especially familial) concern in Fijian communities rather than as a natural and individual concern. The new norm is for a body that is "just right"—neither too fat nor too thin. Girls and their families will pursue an array of methods (including sanctioned use of purgatives) to create and maintain it.

In chapter 8, cultural anthropologist Sarah Trainer presents an ethnographic study of young university students in the United Arab Emirates (UAE), one of the most obese nations in the world. Her analysis mirrors themes from Becker's work in Fiji, detailing the efforts of young, upwardly mobile women and their families to create a body that can bridge both "modern" and "traditional" expectations and pressures. As in Fiji, attaining an appropriate weight is both an individual and family project. Yet women in the UAE also struggle with additional demands to conform to their educated friends' expectations that they achieve the very slim global norms associated with wealth and success. Trainer also details how the women's own standards of an ideal body, coupled with family pressures, lead to unhealthy behaviors. These behaviors likely will carry significant mental and physical costs to their health later in life. Echoing Hruschka's findings in chapter 1, she also details how marriage market sorting around slimmer bodies evolves as UAE families increasingly identify fat bodies as a threat to the chances of a desirable and advantageous marriage.

In the volume conclusion, psychological anthropologist and clinician Rebecca J. Lester and Anderson-Fye revisit the concept of symbolic body capital in light of the varied volume contributions. They discuss the importance of understanding the locally salient qualities of fat, not just quantity, with respect to body capital. Further, drawing on the multilevel analyses presented throughout the volume, they reiterate the *processes* that underlie the work to meet the desired body ideal may be more important than the aesthetic itself. In exploring this idea, they clarify how the chapters together document how the capital of the acceptable body now sits within changing, hybrid, and diversifying markets. These require the complicated challenges of a body presented within multiple markets at once and expanded thinking about the many moral dimensions of body ideals. Then they leave us where all good works should — with an appreciation of the limits of our analytic focus on the economics of fat bodies and with a clearer map of where we need to be heading next as we work to understand what it means to live on an increasingly fat planet.

NOTE

1. Technically, a body mass index (BMI) of over 25 is classified as overweight, and over 30 is classified as obese.

CHAPTER ONE

From Thin to Fat and Back Again
A Dual Process Model of the Big Body Mass Reversal

DANIEL J. HRUSCHKA

Over the past two decades, obesity researchers have consistently identified a reversal in the relationship between body size and economic resources (Dinsa et al. 2012; Hruschka 2012; Monteiro et al. 2004; Sobal and Stunkard 1989; Subramanian et al. 2011). For the poorest 80 percent of contemporary humanity living on less than USD 10 per day, increasing wealth translates to bigger (and fatter) bodies (Hruschka, Hadley, and Brewis 2014). As people become richer, however, this relationship flattens until it reaches a plateau at about USD 3,000–4,000 per capita per year (Dinsa et al. 2012; Monteiro et al. 2004). At this point, men and women diverge in how their body mass index (BMI) relates to economic resources. Male populations remain at this bigger body plateau as they become richer. Female populations, on the other hand, begin a reversal (what I call here the *big body mass reversal*) whereby increasing wealth and income often become statistically associated with *thinner* bodies.

The positive relationship between economic resources and body size experienced by most of contemporary humanity fits a straightforward model of greater consumption in the face of increasing abundance (Brown and Konner 1987; Eaton, Konner, and Shostak 1988; Hruschka 2012). Specifically, as populations have more economic resources to consume calories, they deposit more body mass and become larger. Notably, this explanation does not require invoking any notion of a socially defined ideal body size. Rather, body size may strictly be limited by available resources. Although this resource constraint model works for 80 percent of humanity living on less than USD 10 per day, it breaks down among female populations as they reach sufficiently high levels of economic resources.

Since Sobal and Stunkard (1989) first identified this pattern more than two decades ago, scholars have proposed several theories to explain it. The first class of explanations, found mainly in the nutrition and social determinants of health literatures, assumes that greater wealth provides people the capacity to achieve a society's ideal body size. For example, Sobal and Stunkard (1989, 266) speculated that obesity may be a "sign of health and wealth" in low-income countries but changes from a positive ideal to a stigmatized condition (especially for women) as populations become increasingly wealthy (for one example see Becker, this volume). According to this argument, among poor populations, those with more economic resources can approximate the reigning ideal of obesity more closely. Then, as the ideal reverses with increasing resources, wealthier individuals now use their economic capacity to attain the new thin ideal. This explanation assumes that people actively adjust their body sizes to fit these changing ideals, and that those with the most resources are best able to achieve those ideals. Sobal and Stunkard were agnostic about the specific mechanisms by which people with greater wealth or income were better equipped to approximate reigning body-size ideals. Recently, however, scholars have provided more detailed accounts based on food choice, time constraints on food preparation, and leisure exercise (Hruschka 2012). For example, the energy density hypothesis argues that less-energy-dense foods that protect against obesity (such as vegetables) cost more per calorie. Thus wealthy individuals are best able to consume diets that reduce their weight to fit an ideal of thinness (Drewnowski 2009; Drewnowski and Darmon 2005; Drewnowski and Specter 2004). A related theory focuses on a specific macronutrient—protein—which is thirty to fifty times more costly per calorie than carbohydrates and fats. It also is reported to be more satiating. According to the protein leverage hypothesis, wealthier individuals can purchase foods with higher protein levels. These foods satiate them at lower caloric intakes and prevent them from overconsuming calories (Brooke, Simpson, and Raubenheimer 2010; Simpson and Raubenheimer 2005). A third argument suggests that wealthier individuals have increased access to the kinds of resources—leisure time as well as safe public and private spaces for leisure activity—needed to shape their body size to realize current ideals through physical activity (Gordon-Larsen et al. 2006). Two key assumptions of these theories are that (1) people try to change their body sizes to fit current ideals, and (2) people with greater absolute income and wealth can change their body size by consuming the kinds of foods and engaging in the kinds of physical activity necessary to achieve those ideals.

The second class of body capital–driven theories is closely related to theories described elsewhere in this volume that examine how attractiveness can become a form of exchangeable value (e.g., Edmonds and Mears, McClure, and Taylor). However, some differences among these approaches are worth noting. The bulk of work in demography and economics tests hypotheses with quantitative data and thus relies on common measures of body capital (e.g., BMI) to compare across a wide range of cases. This quantitative approach provides a powerful lens on macrolevel patterns between body capital and economic resources. Until comparable measures of other forms of body capital and attractiveness become available, however, it is impossible to perform the same kind of study with more nuanced notions of beauty and attractiveness based on form, movement, and other factors observed in local descriptions of specific cultural contexts (Anderson-Fye 2004). Hopefully, future work that clearly defines and operationalizes these fine-grained factors for comparison across different contexts will refine our understanding of how bodies viewed from a macrolevel perspective can become valuable and attractive in different cultural contexts. Until that time, BMI, the most commonly used measure of body capital worldwide, provides a first-order approximation of major global trends that complements local descriptions of how body capital shapes access to resources. Even with this one simple measure of bodies, interesting questions and paradoxes arise. In this chapter I seek explanations for the reversal in the relationship between economic resources and BMI as populations become wealthier.

To compare these two classes of theories—resource driven and body capital driven—as explanations for the big body mass reversal, I first detail the key features of this big reversal by offering new analyses of data from low- and middle-income countries and reviewing established patterns in high-income countries. I use novel household-level data from sixty-three countries to document the major dimensions of the big body mass reversal. Finally, I provide predictions from these two theories and assess their fit with established empirical patterns.

OBESITY, BMI, AND SOCIOECONOMIC RESOURCES

Scholars have most commonly identified the reverse gradient using body mass index, based on the assumption that BMI is a good proxy for obesity and excess body fat (Dinsa et al. 2012; Hruschka and Brewis 2013; Hruschka 2012; Monteiro et al. 2004; Sobal and Stunkard 1989; Subramanian et al. 2011). However, body mass confounds two components: "fat mass," or the amount of fat stored in the body, and "fat-free" or "lean mass," which captures the rest of the body's bulk, including bone, muscle, and water. As a result, some cautions must be applied when interpreting BMI as a measure of fat. First, sex differences exist in the meaning of body mass. Women generally have larger quantities of body fat (and greater variability in body fat) than men do. Conversely, men have larger quantities of and variability in lean mass. These differences in body composition mean that body mass is a closer proxy of body fat in women than in men (male R^2 = 0.78 to 0.85, female R^2 = 0.83 to 0.91) and that body mass in men more deeply confounds fat mass and fat-free mass (Hruschka, Rush, and Brewis 2013).

World populations also differ markedly in how much lean mass they start with (their "basal body mass") before accumulating additional body fat. For example, populations that are naturally taller and more slender have less lean mass (and therefore a lower basal body mass) than do populations that are naturally more stocky and muscular. Depending on the measure, populations can differ in their basal body mass by more than 5 kg/m² — the difference between normal weight and obese according to World Health Organization (WHO) guidelines — even though there may be no difference in their levels of fat mass (Hruschka, Hadley, and Brewis 2014; Hruschka, Rush, and Brewis 2013; Rush, Freitas, and Plank 2009; Wells 2009). For example, initial estimates of basal body mass from global surveys suggest that South Asian populations on average have BMI values 4.2 kg/m² lower than native South American populations for the same quantity of body fat (Hruschka et al. 2015; Hruschka, Rush, and Brewis 2013). Combining these populations in the same analyses may lead to inaccurate conclusions regarding economic resources' effects on body fat. If we compared a poor native South American population with a middle-income population of South Asian descent, for example, we may find that they have nearly the same average BMI. From these results, we might infer that wealth has no effect on body fat. However, given the much lower levels of lean mass per height in South Asian populations than in native South American populations, there is likely a large difference in body fat accumulation (about 4.2 kg/m²) that scholars would not detect simply through BMI comparisons between these two populations. In fact, baseline levels of lean mass may vary significantly within countries or regions. Egypt, for example, spans North African and sub-Saharan African populations. Given that North African populations already have more lean mass than sub-Saharan African populations on average, and are also richer, we can anticipate that the North African Egyptian populations will have a higher BMI than the sub-Saharan African Egyptian populations for two reasons: increased wealth *and* higher natural levels of lean mass. This added lean mass among wealthier North African Egyptians would make the effect of wealth look stronger than it actually is. Conversely, if South American populations of largely indigenous ancestry have higher levels of lean mass on average than populations of largely European ancestry, and European ancestry populations are wealthier, these factors could make a wealth–body mass gradient look *weaker* than it actually is. For these reasons, it is important to account for differences in lean mass when comparing across populations (Hruschka et al. 2015; Hruschka, Hadley, and Brewis 2014; Hruschka, Rush, and Brewis 2013).

These sex and population differences are quite remarkable and have led to ample critiques of BMI as a proxy for body fat. However, once we adjust BMI for these sex and population differences, it is a relatively good proxy for total body fat, especially for women (R^2 = 0.83–0.91; Hruschka, Rush, and Brewis 2013).

Socioeconomic status (SES) is even more challenging to measure than body fat. Researchers use many proxies to rank individuals on a social and economic ladder, including education, occupation, income, and wealth. Here I focus on monetary resources—income and wealth—as they can be roughly compared across populations and clear theoretical expectations exist regarding the effects of financial resources on body mass, especially in lower-income populations. That said, I also examine and report the effects of education; researchers have found substantial, but often inconsistent, effects of education on body mass.

KEY DIMENSIONS OF THE BODY MASS REVERSAL

In past studies, researchers have pinpointed the level of wealth or income at which the big body mass reversal occurs by examining the gradient between SES and BMI within countries and then identifying at what national level of wealth or income the gradient turns around (Dinsa et al. 2012; Monteiro et al. 2004; Sobal and Stunkard 1989). One disadvantage of this approach is that it does not provide sufficiently fine-grained data to examine whether this gradient reversal occurs at the same point within regions or across different regions. Here I use a new technique for estimating wealth at the household level in an existing data set of sixty-three low- and middle-income countries (surveys of 656,784 women and 50,742 men). The technique integrates rankings of households by wealth with national-level wealth data so that each household is assigned an estimate of its per capita wealth in the equivalent of US dollars (2011 levels, adjusted for purchasing power; Hruschka, Gerkey, and Hadley 2015). This approach provides sufficiently fine-grained data to offer estimates across and within major world regions (Hadley and Hruschka 2014; Hruschka et al. 2015; Hruschka and Hagaman 2015; Hruschka, Hadley, and Brewis 2014).

To assess the relationship between BMI and wealth in these low- and middle-income countries, I fit a regression predicting BMI from wealth that also permits simultaneous controls for the effect of age, urban residence, education, and breast-feeding on BMI (see the appendix to this chapter). The effect of wealth on BMI becomes stronger as individuals age (Hruschka, Hadley, and Brewis 2014). Thus I limit my analyses to individuals between twenty-five and forty-five years of age who presumably have begun to "enjoy the fruits" of their wealth in terms of increasing adiposity. I also include age in years as a categorical variable to capture nonlinear age increases in BMI. Pregnancy increases BMI, so I exclude pregnant women from these analyses (Hruschka and Hagaman 2015). Given the well-established reduction in BMI with breast-feeding, especially among resource-poor populations, I also control for breast-feeding status (Hruschka and Hagaman 2015). Since a nonlinear relationship exists between ln(wealth) and BMI, I permit the slope relating ln(wealth) to BMI to change at several levels of wealth—USD 500, 2,000, 8,000, and 32,000 per capita. Finally, I stratify analyses by major world region for two reasons: (1) to control for major population differences in basal BMI described earlier, and (2) to examine the consistency of BMI-wealth trajectories across several independent populations.

Here, I examine the following major world regions—Eurasia, South Asia, sub-Saharan Africa, North Africa and the Middle East, Southeast Asia, and South America—using data from the Demographic and Health Surveys (ICF Macro). To examine potential differences in basal body mass among South Americans of predominantly European descent versus predominantly native descent, we also consider these groups as two separate populations. Demographic and Health Surveys collect weight and height on men in far fewer countries, so analyses for men are limited to only two regions—sub-Saharan Africa and South Asia.

Below, I summarize three major observations about the reversal.

Observation 1. The reversal occurs for women at the same level of wealth in most regions of the world. Figure 1.1A shows a consistent relationship between wealth and BMI in female populations from all the world regions examined. Specifically, between USD 500 and 8,000 per capita, average BMI increases by 2 to 4 kg/m². Above USD 8,000 per capita, the relationship between wealth and BMI begins to flatten and then reverses in all world regions, with some

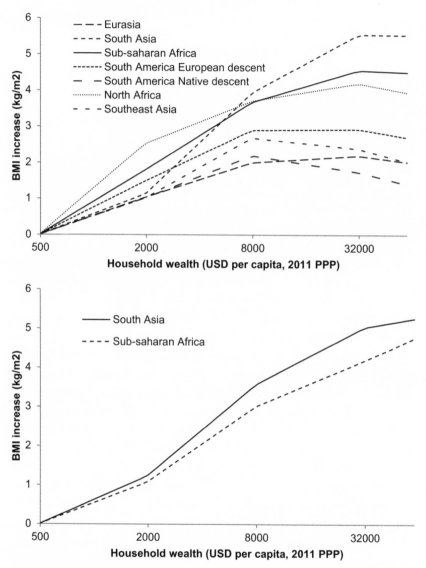

Figure 1.1. Best fit regression model of BMI on wealth in major world regions for (A) females and (B) males.

Table 1.1. Average change in female BMI for every 50 percent increase in household wealth.

Populations	Household wealth per capita (2011 USD)	Increase in BMI for every 50% increase in economic resources
Low- and middle-income countries	500 to 2,000	0.4 kg/m²
	2,000 to 8,000	0.5 kg/m²
	8,000 to 32,000	0.1 kg/m²
	Above 32,000	−0.1 kg/m²
High-income countries	United States (2000s)	−0.3 to −0.6 kg/m²

populations experiencing an earlier turnaround (i.e., Southeast Asian and native South American) than others (i.e., South Asian, sub-Saharan African, and North African). By USD 32,000 per capita, the relationship between wealth and BMI has reversed in women in all populations. Below, I revisit the relationship between wealth and BMI among men.

Table 1.1 shows the average change in female BMI for every 50 percent increase in household wealth at several levels of wealth. This change is most rapid at the lowest wealth categories (0.8 kg/m² for every 50 percent increase in wealth). As populations grow wealthier, the trajectory decelerates and then reverses to a downward slope. We can compare these rates of change with available data from the United States, a country with much higher average wealth per capita, between 1980 and 2000 (Chang and Lauderdale 2005). The US reverse gradient is stronger than the inchoate reversal in the low- and middle-income countries. These results are similar for reverse gradients observed in other countries (Burns 2004). Unfortunately, most published studies of income inequality and obesity only report prevalence of obesity by income, rather than body mass index by income. This limitation makes it difficult to estimate comparable values for more high-income societies.

Observation 2. This reversal does not happen for men. As figure 1.1B illustrates, the reversal does not occur for men in either of the regions—South Asia or sub-Saharan Africa—for which the Demographic and Health Surveys included male anthropometric data. Although the relationship between wealth and BMI attenuates with increasing wealth, it never reverses. This finding of an incipient reversal among women but not men in low- and middle-income countries is consistent with the original results from Sobal and Stunkard as well as more recent studies of the wealth-BMI gradient (Dinsa et al. 2012; Monteiro et al. 2004; Sobal and Stunkard 1989). Moreover, the lack of a reversal in these data cannot be the result of a higher threshold for reversal among men, since men also fail to exhibit a reverse wealth-BMI gradient even in wealthy countries (Dinsa et al. 2012; Monteiro et al. 2004; Sobal and Stunkard 1989).

PREDICTIONS OF THE TWO THEORIES

Now that I have listed key facts about the big body mass reversal, I outline contrasting predictions of the two main classes of theories accounting for the reversal. Since we examine theories aimed at accounting for the reversal, and the reversal occurs among relatively wealthy countries, *these predictions apply to high-income countries.*

Resource-Driven Theories

Income and wealth reduce female body size through a direct effect on food consumption and exercise behavior. Specifically, in high-income societies, women with more household economic resources are more able to achieve the slim body ideal.

Resource-driven prediction 1: within-household correlations. Within a heterosexual married household, household income should correlate with a female spouse's BMI to the degree that she can use that income to achieve a slim ideal. If females have as much or more control over the use of their own income than their spouse's income, the effect of a female's income on BMI should be equal to or greater than the effect of the male spouse's income, but never *less.*

Resource-driven prediction 2: effect among never-married women. The household income–BMI gradient should arise most strongly among never-married women, since they presumably have more control over the use of their entire household income. This idea follows again from the argument that control over the use of economic resources permits women to achieve a lower BMI.

Resource-driven prediction 3: longitudinal changes versus cross-sectional associations. As populations in high-wealth societies acquire more wealth, they should get thinner, as they have more resources to consume thinning foods and to engage in leisure-time exercise. Thus declines in BMI should accompany longitudinal increases in income or wealth.

Body Capital Theories

Women with thinner bodies are able to achieve greater household income and wealth through marriage and labor markets, where a lower BMI is given a premium. Here I layer marriage market and labor market selection factors derived from body capital theories on top of the predictions above.

Body capital prediction 1a: within-household correlations from marriage markets. Within a heterosexual married household, a wife's BMI should be correlated negatively with husband's income but not with her own income. This prediction follows from the argument that thinner women achieve greater income through matching with higher-income spouses.

Body capital prediction 1b: within-household correlations from labor markets. Within a heterosexual married household, a wife's BMI should be correlated negatively with her own income (through labor market selection), but not necessarily her husband's income. This expectation is similar to the prediction from resource-driven theories.

Body capital prediction 2: effect among never-married women. If marriage markets are primarily responsible for the income-BMI gradient, then the household income-BMI gradient should occur primarily among married women, not among those who have never married. This prediction follows from the argument that thinner women acquire greater household resources through a premium in marriage markets.

Prediction 3: longitudinal changes versus cross-sectional associations. As populations acquire more resources, they should get heavier. At any single point in time, however, sorting lower-BMI women into higher income or wealth categories may lead to a reverse BMI-income or BMI-wealth gradient among women.

ASSESSING THE PREDICTIONS

Prediction 1. The first prediction from both theories relates to how the source of household income should (or should not) be related to a spouse's BMI (Averett and Korenman 1996; Averett, Sikora, and Argys 2008; Mukhopadhyay 2008). The most thorough study of this phenomenon to date uses data from the US Panel Study of Income Dynamics from 1999 to 2007 (Chiappori, Oreffice, and Quintana-Domeque 2012; Oreffice and Quintana-Domeque 2010). This study found that among white couples, a 50 percent increase in the husband's income was significantly associated with an average −0.5 to −0.6 kg/m² decrease in the wife's BMI. At the same time, the wife's income had no significant effect on her own BMI (−0.02 kg/m² per 50 percent increase in wife's income). Interestingly, the husband's income has an opposite though weaker effect on his own BMI, with increasing income associated with *increasing* BMI (0.2 to 0.4 kg/m² higher BMI for every 50 percent increase in income). Once again, a wife's income has no relationship to her husband's BMI. The fact that a husband's BMI grows with his own income but not with his wife's may also arise from a selection process in which women are more willing to accept a heavier partner with a higher income (Chiappori, Oreffice, and Quintana-Domeque 2012; Oreffice and Quintana-Domeque 2010). Taken together, these findings suggest that, on average, both women and men in this sample prefer a thinner spouse, with women having a weaker preference for partner thinness than men do. That said, only women on average appear to trade concerns about having a partner with a higher income with one who also is less thin. Estimated from these data, the combination of these preferences would create a wealth-BMI gradient among white women of −0.4 to −0.6 kg/m² for every 50 percent increase in household income. Interestingly, this slope is close to the shape of the reverse gradient observed in white, female US populations (table 1.1). This similarity in the magnitude of effect suggests that this kind of selection process alone could account for the reversal observed in the United States.

Prediction 2. If selection in the marriage market accounts for a large part of the reverse BMI-income gradient among women, then we would also expect that the gradient would be much stronger for married women than for women who have never married. If we examine data from women (ages twenty to forty-nine) from the National Health and Nutrition Examination Survey (NHANES) conducted between 2003 and 2010, we do find such a difference between married and never-married women when a gradient exists (Hruschka 2012; NHANES 2011). For white women (ages twenty-nine to forty-nine), a regression controlling for age shows a strong and significant negative correlation between family income (−0.8 kg/m² per 50 percent increase in income-to-poverty ratio [PIR], 95% CI = −1.0, −0.6, p < 0.0001) but no significant association for never-married women (−0.2 kg/m² per 50 percent increase in PIR, 95% CI = −0.5, 0.1, p > 0.10). We find similar though weaker results for Hispanics/Latinas (−0.4 for married women, p < 0.005 and + 0.2 for never married women, p > 0.10). Consistent with past research about variation in the reverse gradient across ethnic groups (Zhang and Wang 2004), household income had no significant effect on African American women whether married or never married (p < 0.10; see McClure, this volume, for critique of African American females' "exceptionalism," obesity, and body capital). Thus among those groups that exhibit a reverse gradient (non-Hispanic white women and Hispanic/Latina women), the effect occurs among married women, but not among women who have never married.

Prediction 3. The third prediction from both theories involves how changes in economic resources should affect BMI. In a review of available longitudinal evidence, Hruschka shows that in low-, middle-, and high-income countries, an increase in resources has either no effect or a positive effect on BMI, whereas a decrease in resources leads to a reduction or deceleration of growth in BMI (Forde et al. 2011; Hruschka 2012). For example, incomes rose for all income deciles in the United States in the latter half of the twentieth century (Jones and Weinberg 2000). Corresponding with this increase was a historical *increase* in BMI among all income groups (Chang and Lauderdale 2005). However, at any cross-sectional time slice during that period, women with lower incomes had on average higher BMIs (Chang and Lauderdale 2005). Analyses of cross-sectional data using instrumental variable approaches show that observed correlations between financial hardship and obesity among women are not likely a direct result of financial hardship but due to confounding by unobservable variables (Averett and Smith 2013). Few natural experiments randomly manipulate income, making it difficult to examine the true causal relationship between increasing resources and BMI. However, researchers recently made use of a glitch in the US Social Security system that gave people born between 1915 and 1917 a higher benefit than those born earlier or later. Researchers used this anomaly as a natural quasi-experiment to examine how much artificially inflated Social Security benefits affected body mass index. They found that a USD 1,000 increase in annual Social Security benefits from this glitch had no significant effect on current BMI (+0.01 kg/m²; Cawley, Moran, and Simon 2010). Thus there are few if any examples of populations becoming thinner as they acquire more resources. Rather, as populations accrue more resources, they often (but not always) gain weight. At any one slice in time, however, wealthier individuals, specifically women, may have lower body mass than poorer individuals (Hruschka 2012).

Prediction 4. The body capital–driven theory relying on labor market mechanisms also makes a unique prediction about the effect of body size on earnings. Over the last decade, a wealth of observational studies have documented how heavier women in wealthy countries experience a wage penalty as well as greater challenges finding employment in a range of high-income countries, including Germany (Caliendo and Lee 2013), Ireland (Mosca 2013), China (Pan, Qin, and Liu 2012), and the United States (Han, Norton, and Powell 2011; Han, Norton, and Stearns 2009). In addition, studies in Germany and the United States that separate fat mass and lean mass indicate that there is a wage penalty specifically for adiposity, whereas there is actually a slight wage premium for lean mass (e.g., more muscular individuals earn higher wages than their less muscular peers). The counterposed effects of these two components of body mass may explain the relative lack of association between wages and body mass index among men (Bozoyan and Wolbring 2011; Wada and Tekin 2010). Although there does appear to be a wage penalty for obesity, studies that attempt to estimate its magnitude suggest that it is much less forceful in sorting individuals than the marriage market. Specifically, although a 0.5 kg/m^2 reduction in a woman's BMI is associated with an average increase of 50 percent in a spouse's income, that same reduction in BMI is associated with an increase of only about 1 percent in one's own income (Han, Norton, and Powell 2011). Thus marriage markets in wealthy countries appear to be *fifty times stronger* than labor markets in their ability to generate the big body mass reversal.

DISCUSSION

Researchers have proposed two kinds of hypotheses to account for the big body mass reversal as populations grow richer. Resource-driven theories argue that increasing economic resources give people greater capacity to reduce their body size through exercise and the consumption of thinning foods. In contrast, body capital theories argue that in wealthy countries, women with thinner bodies can achieve income premiums in both marriage and labor markets. Several lines of evidence presented here are consistent with predictions of the body capital theories but inconsistent with the resource-driven theories.

First, economic resources in heterosexual married households are not uniformly associated with a wife's BMI. Indeed, her BMI is significantly associated with her husband's income but not her own. This pattern suggests that instead of household resources permitting a thinner body, a thinner body for women on this sample can, on average, attract more household resources. Second, increasing household resources are associated with reduced BMI among married women in a representative US sample but not among women who have never married. These findings suggest that achieving greater income through marriage—rather than some generic effect of income on BMI—is a key factor in creating the reverse gradient. Third, longitudinal data in which individuals experience income gains or losses do not support the idea that declining resources lead to increasing BMI. Rather, with increasing resources a population will tend to accrue body mass or stay constant but rarely reduce BMI. This recurring finding is consistent with a resource-driven theory that increases in wealth drive increasing body mass. However, it is clearly *not* consistent with resource-driven theories that explain the big body mass reversal by increasing resources leading to *reductions* in BMI. Finally, among the two possible market mechanisms proposed to match thinner bodies with greater economic resources, marriage markets appear to create a much stronger gradient—and one of comparable magnitude with the gradient observed in the United States and Australia.

Taken together, this diverse evidence suggests that two processes likely create the big body mass reversal observed among women as populations become increasingly wealthy. The first process is most visible in low- and middle-income countries. As populations gain more economic resources, they consume more calories than they use, and they gain weight. As the data here and in other sources demonstrate, the effect of economic resources is strongest for the poorest and flattens as populations grow wealthier. If this process worked alone, then there should be no reversal in the trend toward increasing body size among women or men (see dotted line, fig. 1.2). Indeed, we observe a slow leveling off of body size among men (fig. 1.1B). In the case of women, however, a second process reverses the direction of causation as well as the relationship between body size and economic resources (fig. 1.1A). Instead of more resources leading to bigger bodies, bigger bodies make it more difficult to acquire resources through marriage (and, to a lesser extent, wage labor). It is not clear whether this sorting process occurs in low- and middle-income countries, but strong evidence exists that it does occur in high-income countries (Averett and Korenman 1996; Chiappori, Oreffice, and Quintana-Domeque 2012; Mukhopadhyay 2008; Oreffice and Quintana-Domeque 2010). If this body capital process were the only one affecting the wealth-BMI relationship, then the gradient would look like the dashed line in figure 1.2. When these two processes act together, they create the observed reverse gradient (solid line in fig. 1.2), with the first, resource-driven process having the biggest influence at low income levels and

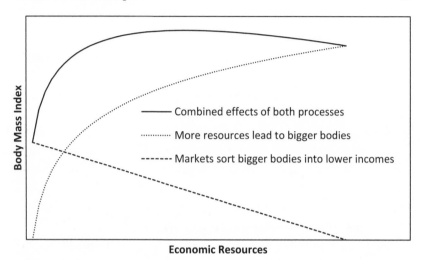

Figure 1.2. Two processes and how they would combine to create a reverse gradient.

the second, body capital-driven process having a relatively larger influence at high income levels. Whether or not the second process operates in low-income countries merits study (Thomas and Strauss 1997), but it would need to be extremely strong compared to what exists in the United States and high-income countries to change the overall qualitative trajectory.

It is important to note that this dual-process model does not require conscious effort to change body size, which is consistent with the difficulties most people face in controlling their body sizes (Kassirer and Angell 1998; Becker, this volume). Rather, the first process only requires that people consume more in the face of increasing resources, and the second process only requires that marriage markets sort thinner women into wealthier households.

The dual-process model described here is consistent with a range of cross-sectional and longitudinal observations about the relationships between income and body mass in both low- and high-income countries. It also raises interesting questions that have not been explored with empirical studies. For example, in high-income countries, marriage markets appear to sort thinner individuals into higher income categories. However, in poorer countries, the strength and direction of this sorting mechanism is unclear. Marriage markets' influence would depend on the strength of hypergamy on attractiveness and on the degree to which different levels of BMI are considered more or less attractive. Given the dominant role of increasing resources in driving BMI in low-income settings, such variation is unlikely to change the general predictions of the model. However, it may help us understand precisely how much economic resources affect weight gain in low-income settings.

These findings do not mean that women prefer only higher incomes in spouses and men only prefer thinner women. These are average results explaining a population-level phenomenon in wealthy countries, and they mask a great deal of variation between individuals in their preferences and goals. Moreover, evidence from the above studies indicates both women and men in the United States prefer spouses with thinner bodies and the real asymmetry revolves around gender differences in concerns about spousal income. These variations also do not necessarily reflect innate biological tendencies. Indeed, it is possible that these asymmetries in preferences emerge from an already-unequal system—that is, men on average have access to higher salaries for the same effort. It would be interesting to examine how a society's gender equality in wages influences the reverse income–BMI gradient by changing the trade-offs in marriage markets. Specifically, if asymmetries in the labor market influence mate preferences, which in turn influence the income-BMI gradient, then we would expect countries with greater gender equality in income and greater equality in access to wage markets to have a weaker (or nonexistent) reverse income–BMI gradient among women.

Finally, it is important to note that body capital can come in many forms, and that the current focus on BMI is aimed at a specific BMI-related puzzle—the big body mass reversal. As researchers identify other ways of assessing attractiveness that permit macrolevel analyses as described here, we will encounter new, interesting puzzles that can be explored with similar approaches. These examinations will further refine and structure our models of how people manage their bodies with available resources and how in turn these managed bodies provide new avenues for upward mobility.

APPENDIX: ADDITIONAL RESULTS
FROM REGRESSION MODELS

The regression model shows an expected negative effect of breast-feeding on BMI among females (−0.1 to −0.6 BMI units depending on world region). There is a positive effect of urban residence among females (0.0 to 1.3 BMI units depending on world region), and among South Asian males (0.1), but a significant negative effect for sub-Saharan males (−0.3). Education has significant but widely varying effects on BMI, showing a positive effect in South Asia (+0.4 for primary and +0.2 for higher among females, and +0.3 and +0.5 among males) and sub-Saharan Africa (+0.7 and +0.4 for females and +0.7 and +0.5 for males) and a negative effect in East Asia (−0.3 and −1.1), South America (−0.1 and −1.2 for European descent and −0.2 and −1.2 for native descent), Eurasia (−0.2 and −1.2), and North Africa (−0.6 and −1.8).

CHAPTER TWO

Managing Body Capital in the Fields of Labor, Sex, and Health

ALEXANDER EDMONDS AND ASHLEY MEARS

In many domains, attractiveness carries a value that can potentially be exchanged for other benefits. This valuing of the body can create new opportunities in such realms as fashion, service work, and sexual relationships, but it also can contribute to body commodification and pressures to change body shape and appearance. In this chapter we discuss the uses and limits of the concept of body capital in understanding how attractiveness is valued, exchanged, and managed in consumer capitalism.

The body capital concept implies that attractiveness is a resource that belongs to an individual that can be exchanged for other resources. However, we stress that capital is a metaphor, and like all metaphors, it foregrounds some matters and obscures others. Whereas some economists have measured gains from body capital (e.g., Hammermesh 2011), we concentrate on how social conditions determine its value and enable its exchange. We draw on a range of empirical examples, including our respective ethnographic studies of plastic surgery in Brazil (Edmonds 2010, 2013) and global fashion modeling and highly exclusive (VIP) nightclubs (Mears 2011, 2014).

Several works in sociology and anthropology recently discussed body capital (e.g., Bernstein 2007) and related terms—among them *physical capital* (Shilling 1993), *aesthetic capital* (Anderson et al. 2010), *sexual capital* (Edmonds 2010; Green 2011), *pugilistic capital* (Wacquant 1995), and *girl capital* (Mears 2014). These terms can be regarded as the conceptual offspring of Bourdieu's (1984, 84) analysis of "embodied cultural capital," although not all of this work retains his critique of class domination—a key issue to which we will return. These studies draw on empirical research involving quite different social phenomena, such as boxing, sex work, and modeling. They also are concerned with different qualities of the body, including height, beauty, or erotic skills. Nevertheless, the works reveal a shared interest in comprehending how such qualities become resources that can be exchanged for other benefits.

Such exchanges take place in "markets"—another economic concept frequently associated with body capital. We put the term in quotation marks because we are talking about markets not only in the conventional sense (e.g., labor or beauty service markets) but also in the looser sense of dating or marriage markets. Of course, these markets are not all equivalent (Martin and George 2006). The exchange of labor for a wage is a more direct and socially regulated transaction than is, say, the exchange of love and material resources. Even so, the idea of a market for body capital is useful in that it can shed light on the pressures and opportunities that surround appearance in various, often overlapping, domains of life. We focus on how body capital is valued and exchanged in the fields of health, labor, and sexuality. In addition, we explore the implications these practices have for social inequality.

The market metaphor indicates that the "fair price" of attractiveness is determined by supply and demand. However, one weakness of many body capital analyses is that the concept is framed exclusively as an individual possession without considering the conditions in which it is considered valuable. For example, Hakim (2010) urges women to cultivate erotic capital as a means of personal empowerment that can remedy gender inequality (see Green 2013 for a critique). We argue that attractiveness is a partly inherited quality of a person that, to some extent, yields benefits that do not conform to class, ethnic, or other social hierarchies. However, we also analyze the power relations that help determine the value of this resource and govern the "terms" of its conversion. The benefits derived from a person's body capital can be appropriated by others. Moving beyond the personal-advantage perspective, we consider how benefits from the valuation and circulation of bodily capital are distributed unequally in social systems (Mears 2014).

Finally, we discuss how this analysis can illuminate practices that seek to *manage* body shape and fat. Much discussion of the global growth in weight-related health problems has focused on lifestyle and biological causes of obesity (see Brewis 2011). Although health is one important domain in which fat is valued, however, it is not the only one. Fat has varying economic, aesthetic, and moral values. For example, body fat may be valued in one way in a labor market that rewards thinness, another way in an erotic field, and yet a third way in a social environment that attributes moral failings to overweight people. Although health and fitness are often seen as a precondition of beauty, many sexual and aesthetic ideals go "against" health: the pale consumptive of nineteenth-century Europe, the Chinese bound foot, and the global fashion model's extreme thinness (Edmonds 2013). Such versions of beauty are valued partly due to their scarcity (as with many economic goods) but also because of their removal from everyday concerns with production and reproduction. In contemporary efforts to manage body capital, tensions can emerge between health rationales and other concerns that involve social status, economic pressures, and the erotic imagination.

Analyzing body capital thus can highlight that weight management often is much more than a health issue. Public health campaigns against fat feed—and feed off—other pressures and aspirations. This trend is particularly meaningful as body capital becomes a more salient quality of the person in labor and sexual fields. Understanding how fat is valued in different social domains is important for several reasons. Perhaps most important, this knowledge carries significant implications for health: many practices to reduce weight in fact have considerable risks, whereas fat stigma has psychological and social consequences that can potentially harm well-being and health (Brewis, Hruschka, and Wutich 2011; Brownell et al. 2005).

ATTRACTIVENESS AS A FORM OF VALUE

Does it make sense to speak of attractiveness as a persisting *quality of the person*—as opposed to a transient perception dependent on changing social circumstances? One problem with the body capital concept is that human beauty and ugliness have multiple effects of attraction and repulsion that are difficult to capture with an economic metaphor. Attractiveness seems to comprise a range of qualities, some to do with the body's physical attributes, some with expressions of mind or spirit, and some with skills and tastes. There is also an ineffable aspect to attractiveness; its descriptions often use energy metaphors, for example, radiance, warmth, or coolness.[1] The beautiful person fascinates in part because gazing at him or her can transport the viewer from utilitarian or pragmatic concerns (Scarry 2001).

Although there is undeniably a subjective aspect to beauty, perceptions of attractiveness nevertheless can be shared across national, class, ethnic, and other boundaries—perhaps more than judgments of "good" style or taste. Like height or hair color, words denoting an attractive person often are used in everyday speech to identify an unknown individual (e.g., "he's a good-looking guy"). On the other hand, the perception of attractiveness can be contextual and shaped by other qualities of the person, such as class or ethnic markers, charm, and so forth. However much the good-looking person may spark admiration, desire, or other affects, the valuing of beauty occurs in social and historical conditions often beyond the individual's control—or even awareness. Whereas attractiveness is a quality that potentially confers benefits, power relations determine the actual value of body capital and when it can—or must—be exchanged.

BODY CAPITAL AND SOCIAL HIERARCHY

This notion of body capital builds on the three forms of capital analyzed by Pierre Bourdieu (1984, 1986): economic, social, and cultural. In his framework, *cultural capital* refers to taste, knowledge, or skills that are valued by a particular class segment. *Social capital* derives from networks of influence and support. One of Bourdieu's main aims—not always present in later uses of his work— was to analyze how classes reproduce themselves through the exchange of different forms of capital.

Yet the concept also stands in tension with this trio. Since attractiveness can help confer wealth it might seem to be a variant of Bourdieu's notion of embodied cultural capital. For example, researchers report higher salaries for men above average height (Harper 2000). Attractiveness thus resembles forms of cultural capital, such as education, in that it can be converted into economic benefits. However, attractiveness is not simply a variant of cultural capital but is a distinct form of value not reducible to other qualities of the person.

Bourdieu himself seems to acknowledge this point when he refers to an anomaly in class reproduction. For Bourdieu, the body "is the most indisputable materialization of class taste" (1984, 190). Class-based bodily skills and dispositions—what Bourdieu called the *habitus*—are internalized and embodied at an early age and thus become natural or second nature (101). However, later in the same work he concedes that

> the logic of social heredity sometimes endows those least endowed . . .
> with the rarest bodily properties, such as beauty (sometimes "fatally"
> attractive, because it threatens the other hierarchies, and, conversely,
> sometimes denies the "high and mighty" the bodily attributes of their
> position, such as height or beauty). (193)

Bourdieu suggests here that some physical qualities—such as beauty or height—are not valued or distributed according to other social hierarchies. Those who are endowed with high levels of economic, social, or cultural capital—or even all three—nevertheless may be unattractive or short; conversely, both men and women can possess exceptional beauty regardless of their social origin (Edmonds 2010).

This comment provides a rich opportunity to analyze power relations surrounding attractiveness. Most social science and humanities scholarship has viewed attractiveness as an illustration of other forms of social inequality. That women are judged by appearance more than men reflects patriarchal relations (e.g., Wolf 1991). Aesthetic hierarchies in multiracial societies mirror larger racial domination (Kaw 1993). These critiques are important, but they do not describe fully the significance of attractiveness for social life (or social science). Instead, they tend to reduce beauty norms—and the social responses to them—to a mechanical reflection of other forms of power, emptying this domain of anything specific to it. Ethnic "others," whether exoticized or denigrated, still can be seen as attractive. Aesthetic markers of status are not always congruent with class indicators. Attractiveness is also a dimension of the self; sometimes it is a resource that actors use in negotiating the social boundaries that otherwise limit their lives. Body capital can reinforce existing relations of domination but also can undermine other systems of status marking. For black Americans the aesthetic valuing of skin color can have greater consequences for stratification than racial classification alone (Monk 2014).

At the same time, perceptions of attractiveness *are* simultaneously shaped by class, racial, and patriarchal inequalities. These power dynamics become more evident through detailed analysis of the specific "fields" in which body capital is valued and exchanged (Martin and George 2006). Bourdieu (1993) used the metaphor of fields (with origins in military and natural science) to show that valuing is a contested activity. Each field has its own "rules of the game"; what is valued in one domain is not always valued in another. In the field of cultural production, for example, some forms of "good taste" have a value that does not translate to the field of global finance.

Sexual fields too have their own rules. For example, the erotic capital exchanged by gay black men in New York City (Green 2011) has a different value from that employed by Chinese women in relationships with foreigners (Farrer 2010). Women are penalized at the workplace for being "too" attractive far more than men are. Females also pay a higher penalty than men for being overweight (Hammermesh 2011; Green 2013, 154). Appearance is a domain of discipline for women more than men, reflecting gendered inequalities and women's greater vulnerability to eating disorders (Wolf 1991; Bartky 1990).

We build on Bourdieu's analysis of how social inequalities influence conversions of capital but also argue that attractiveness is a partly inherited form of value not wholly determined by other status markers. We develop this approach with some empirical examples of how body capital operates within the entangled fields of labor and sexual relationships.

Body Capital in Labor Fields

One obvious field in which appearance becomes a form of capital is labor. Economists have shown that attractive male and female workers (according to anonymous observers) earn substantially more income than average-looking workers (Hammermesh 2011). This seems to be an example of a relatively straightforward exchange of capital for financial reward. Yet although this beauty effect has been found in diverse labor sectors, the "rules" that govern the value of attractiveness—and the terms of exchange—vary.

In fashion modeling, for example, body shape and appearance are valued according to field-specific rules. Drawing on long-term fieldwork in this industry, Mears (2011) found that the values of bodies are polarized between two segments of the field, editorial fashion and commercial fashion. Editorial models generally earn less money but have higher status through ties to prestigious fashion houses and magazines; commercial models, in contrast, earn consistently high wages but are lower status in the industry; as a result, they have far fewer chances to become superstars than do the editorial models.[2]

What counts as body capital—or in industry jargon, a desirable "look"—varies systematically in each segment of the field. Models in editorial work have a rarer, "edgy" look; their higher status (and lower pay) comes in part from the smaller audience of fashion insiders who have the codified knowledge to appreciate their idiosyncratic looks. Field outsiders sometimes refer to these models as "strange looking" or even "ugly." Commercial looks, widely described as "classic" or "soft," stand in sharp contrast to edgy editorial ones. They are more appropriate for lower-status catalogue work, which in the long run can damage the brand of the model. Although fashion has often been critiqued for promoting narrow beauty ideals, internal differentiation within the industry between model looks is actually crucial for conversions of bodily capital. (Surprisingly, the "personality" of the model also is important for an individual's industry success.)

The larger political and economic context of the industry matters for such conversions too. The physical type of the fashion model is genetically rare, which helps establish value; however, this value also changes over time. For example, the rise of more aggressive scouting efforts, as well as the opening of new markets in Russia and Eastern Europe, has led to a surge in women aspiring to model. As a result of increased supply in a formerly rare type of "beauty," the value of this form of bodily capital has declined in recent years, with models' wages dropping across the field. Fashion's criteria of physical attractiveness are particularly exacting, but attractiveness also functions as an exchangeable resource in other industries. For example, in some retail settings, employees are called "models," allowing workers to tap into the fantasy of the model life (Williams and Connell 2010).

The valuing of body capital is often visible in practices to *manage* appearance. Edmonds (2010) became interested in how appearance is valued while conducting ethnographic fieldwork on plastic surgery in Brazil, now the world's largest market for cosmetic procedures. Some public hospitals with plastic surgery residency programs go so far as to offer free cosmetic procedures. Price competition among surgeons, along with the expansion of consumer credit, have given Brazilians from a wide range of socioeconomic backgrounds access to cosmetic surgery.

Both surgeons and psychologists who screened potential patients were disturbed by the many candidates who expected surgeries to resolve life problems beyond the medical domain. Both working-class and wealthier patients spoke of aspirations and anxieties related to labor markets. Telenovelas, pop songs, and news media in Brazil and Latin America have portrayed plastic surgery—widely referred to simply as *plástica*—as a means to achieve fame and wealth. Many women seeking jobs in Brazil's vibrant culture and entertainment industries as models, actresses, and dancers saw plástica as an essential "career move." A producer from Globo, Brazil's largest television network, told a *morena* (brown, mixed) woman that she should have surgery on her nose because a thinner nose increased her opportunities to be cast in a greater variety of roles. More surprisingly, many poorer patients who performed low-income service work as secretaries, receptionists, vendors, and hotel staff said they hoped to find new employment or life opportunities with cosmetic surgery. Others spoke of fears of getting fired due to an aged, "ugly," or not sufficiently white appearance.

In service work, traits such as youth and attractiveness can become hiring criteria or add value to transactions. Although paid domestic service remains remarkably widespread among women in urban peripheries, many Brazilians try to avoid such work. For them, the most viable option is a job in the growing service sector (Goldenberg 2000). Color barriers, however, continue to operate in labor markets. Discrimination is illegal, but some employers favor workers with a *boa aparência* (good appearance), often understood to mean "white or comparative lightness." Color, as well as the body itself, are often seen as malleable or plastic in Brazil (Edmonds and Sanabria 2014). Beauty techniques, such as skin lighteners and hair straighteners, can change how color and status are ascribed. In these circumstances body capital—comprising a mix of traits, such as youth, beauty, and relative lightness of skin—can be perceived as a means to mitigate social exclusion, compete in service markets, or even attain fame and wealth, as in the widespread social fantasy of becoming a fashion model (Edmonds 2010).

Body Capital in Sexual Fields

Whereas surgeons positioned plástica as a means of psychological healing, patients often envisioned the body as a valuable but precarious resource that required management to compete or thrive in labor—as well as sexual—fields. Some women Edmonds (2010) interviewed discussed appearance as an important resource in what they called the "market" of dating (*namorando*.) Flavia, for example, commented that women are "traded" in a market in which age and attractiveness are principal sources of value. She saw plastic surgery as a means to offset the depreciation of body capital caused by aging. Attractiveness can thus be envisioned explicitly as a fungible asset that requires maintenance.

The idea that a market exists for sexual relationships and marriage is not recent. Marx argued that true sentiment was impossible in bourgeois marriage because the practice of the dowry meant that women were valued according to their families' wealth. A market of relationships or marriage could be said to operate when desirable and undesirable qualities in partners are "measured" (by each other or by marriage brokers) and traded. For example, wealth can be exchanged for social pedigree or attractiveness, and attractiveness can compensate for poverty or "mask" the lack of personal qualities such as virtue. Sexual selection, in these terms, is a "rating and dating complex" (Waller 1937).

Sexual and marriage markets exist in a range of historical conditions, but transformations in consumer capitalism can create markets in which body capital is particularly important. Activities such as sports, dance, beach going, fashion, and beautification all draw attention to the body, making it a more central domain of identity (Edmonds 2010). Norms such as "elective sexuality," "plastic sexuality," or "serial monogamy," which delink sex from the reproductive imperative or heterosexual marriage, can make attractiveness a more important quality in relationships assumed to be transient (Giddens 1993). The decline of the moral ideal of female sexual modesty and rise of postfeminist "sex-positive" norms may create more freedom and choice but also more competition. Delayed marriage and the rise in divorce and separation, trends across the industrialized world (Castells 1997), mean that more people are single and potentially dating for longer periods of the life cycle. More partner choice may lead to people placing more value on physical appearance as men and women compete in larger pools of potential partners.

The value of body capital functions differently depending on the field, sexual or labor. For example, whereas romantic partners more discreetly exchange beauty for compensation like gifts or "treats" (Piess 1986), the bodies of retail workers are carefully selected and groomed with various degrees of explicit commodification (Nickson et al. 2001). We argue that work and sexual fields— despite differences between them—often overlap. Service work can transform youth and sexual allure into job assets, creating pleasures as well as vulnerabilities to sexual objectification and harassment (Warhurst and Nickson 2009; Williams and Connell 2010). In Brazil, aspiring models and actresses complain of the "sofa audition," the expectation that sex must be exchanged for a role in an ad or television drama (Edmonds 2010).

In the highly exclusive (or VIP) club party scene Mears (2014) studied, leisure often overlaps with labor and can become conflated with transactional sex. Fashion models are recruited to participate in high-end party scenes because their body capital (youth, height, beauty, and whiteness) is essential to the clubs' economic success (see also Grazian 2008). However, models also must differentiate themselves from other women in the scene who participate in transactional sex.

The VIP scene is of course elite, requiring substantial money, entrepreneurial skills, or genetically rare forms of body capital to participate. However, other fields and subcultures also raise complex questions about autonomy and commodification in the exchange of body capital. Online dating—a diversified, global field—can facilitate conversions of body capital in that it permits the rapid scanning of images and information about body shape and ethnicity (Logan 2012). Some sites, such as Seeking Arrangements, specialize in niches that verge on commercial sex work, and sex work itself has become more mainstream in some regions. Bernstein (2007) found that middle-class sex work includes not just cash-for-sex transactions but also complex exchanges involving gifts, emotional intimacy, tuition, or rent.

The Internet and ease of travel also foster transnational dating scenes where body capital figures centrally. "Mail-order bride" companies enable men to find partners younger and more attractive than they might otherwise. In "romance tourism," both men and women exchange their greater economic and cultural capital for sex or romance with younger or more attractive partners or those who offer authentic holiday experiences (Wiss 2006). In postsocialist countries, sexual fields often undergo changes that facilitate body capital exchange. For example, in China various forms of transactional sex have become more salient as "call girls" publish online diaries and the mistress becomes a status symbol for businessmen (Osburg 2011). Body *management* practices also often grow rapidly as countries embrace consumer capitalism: once a suppressed "bourgeois" practice in the Maoist era, plastic surgery is an often-normalized beauty practice in China today (Brownell 2005).

WHO OWNS BODY CAPITAL?

These examples of how body capital is exchanged in different fields raise the crucial question of ownership, a point often sidestepped in economistic accounts of human capital. Who "owns" this form of capital? Many fields and subcultures could be said to be undemocratic in that they reward those who are young or attractive but lack "moral" or other positive personal qualities. Yet physical attractiveness and youth can interfere with the class and color hierarchies that otherwise prevail. The value of symbolic status markers can be partially suppressed when relationships are based primarily on physical qualities. Sexual fields can provide opportunities where body capital can potentially, though often transiently, subvert structures of inequality. Ownership, then, seems to lie within the body endowed with this capital.

On the other hand, framing embodied capital as an individual property neglects the conditions enabling the appropriation of capital (Mears 2014). In fashion, models get some financial and symbolic reward from their body capital, but (largely male) owners of luxury fashion conglomerates often profit even more. In many sex and service industries, much of the value of women's bodies benefits men, who make up the majority of owners and managers in these industries (Sanders and Hardy 2012). Women's bodily capital is indeed valuable—but valuable to *whom* remains an important question.

Consider the case of the global VIP party circuit. Based on fieldwork at high-end parties in New York, Miami, and the French Riviera, Mears (2014) analyzed how women's bodily capital is transformed into *girl capital*, a resource men appropriate to generate status, profit, and social connections in the exclusive global leisure circuit. VIP clubs are exclusive nightclubs offering "bottle service" to the global "jet set." Patrons rent tables and buy whole bottles of alcohol at prices ranging from $250 to $5,000. The key actors in the VIP party space are "whales" (wealth club clients), "party promoters" (largely male brokers who recruit women to clubs), and "girls" (women who are not paid to be there but receive gifts of free entrance, drinks, and meals). These women are young (sixteen to twenty-five), thin, tall, and typically (though not exclusively) white. They are ubiquitously called "girls," regardless of age. Exploiting the correlation between attractiveness and status (Webster and Driskell 1983), clubs and their promoters want beautiful female populations of a specifically rare sort in the form of fashion models. In this field, the model body denotes a space as elite. Physical looks take primacy over other embodied cues of class such as accent or comportment.

Party promoters, mostly male brokers, use gifts, charm, friendship, discipline, and "strategic intimacies"—relationships grounded in explicit economic interests—to recruit women to come to clubs, whose presence lures "whales," the wealthy clients. Some women enjoy the parties and the perks and social networks that go with them. However, in the long run, men's gains are likely to be far greater than women's. The most common benefits for women—drinks, dinners, trips, and housing—are not transferrable or asset growing, unlike the revenue they help generate for the clubs and their owners. Promoters use the presence of the girls to gain access to the VIPs, to signal their own status, and to create an environment in which significant business ties are built. Girl capital also brings revenues for the club and its staff. This system of traffic in women enables class consolidation among men in the global elite while reproducing gender inequality at the top of the social class hierarchy.

In the VIP club case, women's participation is framed as leisure; sex-for-money transactions are discouraged. However, both promoters and women also do meticulous "boundary work" (Lamont and Molnar 2002) to differentiate their activities from pimping and sex work, which would devalue girl capital. Actors make careful distinctions between "girls," who voluntarily go with promoters to the clubs to "have fun," and various other categories of women, including "bottle girls" (who serve alcohol), "table girls" (who are paid cash to sit at tables), and "bitches" (understood as women who exchange sex for gifts or money). Such symbolic boundaries demarcating labor from leisure actually perpetuate the unequal value of women's body capital, since women are culturally prohibited from capitalizing on the exchange value of their own bodies; doing so would risk association with sex work.

This analysis of the VIP club scene highlights that sexual and labor fields can become intertwined, augmenting the risks and opportunities that flow from conversions of body capital. When studying the value of bodies, it is important to consider ownership and appropriation, including the unequal opportunity structures that enable only some to harness the long-term value of body capital.

TECHNIQUES TO MANAGE BODY SHAPE AND WEIGHT

In contemporary consumer capitalism many people are put into situations—for longer periods of their lives—where they confront opportunities and pressures to exchange body capital. We now discuss some of the ways people *manage* body capital in these social conditions.

Public concern has been rising regarding practices to control body weight. A wide range of such practices exist: from eating disorders to medically supervised weight-loss surgery, from beauty work to medical cosmetic surgery, from healthy exercise to unhealthy body building and steroid use. Of course these practices have quite different rationales and it might seem odd to lump them together. In fact, much medical and media discussion aims to *distinguish* between body practices that are healthy and those that are harmful (though expert knowledge frequently changes). Miracle diets and pills are generally "bad." Moderate exercise is almost always "good." Beauty work helps self-esteem but can have health risks. However, although there are important differences in these body practices, they can all be incited by the valuing of bodies. It is thus important to consider how efforts to manage body weight are not only motivated by health concerns, but also respond to diverse life pressures and opportunities.

In fashion modeling, even a small amount of body fat can harm the model's career, leading to disordered eating behaviors among models pursuing "size zero" bodies. This struggle is increasingly difficult over the course of a model's career as he or she moves from a teenage, pre-pubescent body into an adult body (Mears 2011). Two centuries ago, a full-figured female body connoted privilege; today thinness signifies qualities such as self-control, wealth, modernity, and a remove from utilitarian activities of mothering or work. In the contemporary United States and Europe, abundant flesh in the female body is associated with lower-class status and sexual availability, whereas the "high-end" look is embodied by thinness—as evidenced in sites ranging from fashion (Mears 2011) to strip clubs (Trautner 2005).

The capacity of fat to become imbued with aesthetic and material (and not just health) value has important implications for global efforts to reduce obesity-related disease. Many countries in the developing world are experiencing an epidemiological transition whereby noncommunicable diseases, such as diabetes and heart disease, are causing more harm than infectious diseases. As a result, public-health campaigns are focusing more on lifestyle and diet—in some cases by featuring images of fit, thin, and sexy consumers. Such campaigns can conflate "health" with other status markers, such as a modern or middle-class lifestyle or even relative lightness of skin. Efforts to promote healthier eating may not be relevant to local practices or may be invested with class meaning, as Susan Reynolds Whtye's (2014) work in Uganda showed. Media images of smart families eating "health foods" such as fruit yogurt and oatmeal embed health messages in local status dynamics. Too much body fat can indicate low status, whereas "healthiness"—as defined by global campaigns—can signify a modern, middle-class identity. Efforts to change body shape can have harmful health or economic consequences when significant household resources are spent on imported (but not necessarily healthier) foods or dietary supplements.

We have argued that pressures to control body weight come from many domains beyond public health. Indeed, the news media, fashion, and self-help industries seem to reiterate messages about the need and ways to lose or manage weight (Saguy 2013). This convergence in valuing thinness could be praised because of the health benefits weight loss can have. However, the public health message to control weight through lifestyle can fuel other body management techniques that ultimately may harm health. Anorexia is sometimes seen as a distorted mirror to the "good" health message to be thin. Following exposure to Western media, eating disorders have risen in the non-Western world. This trend shows that thinness is not just a health ideal but also involves other social messages (Anderson-Fye 2004; Becker, this volume). The difficulty in *treating* eating disorders—as well as obesity—suggests that body weight and appearance are often highly charged with moral, emotional, and aesthetic significance.

Health-oriented management of fat can also become entangled with sexual and aesthetic rationales for changing body shape, which also can pose health risks. For example, one reason plastic surgery has become so prevalent and acceptable in Brazil is that it is seen often as a health or hygienic practice; as a result, it is increasingly integrated into mainstream women's health care. Cosmetic surgeries become morally authorized when they seek to attain body ideals that are promoted by mainstream obstetricians and gynecologists as well as in public health messages. This blurring of health and aesthetics is illustrated by names of new medical specialties, such as "aesthetic medicine" or "aesthetic endocrinology," which combine health care with beautification and erotic enhancement (Edmonds 2013).

Health and aesthetics can also become knotted with controversial weight-loss surgeries. In the United States, bariatric surgery is an elective procedure. Officially it has the health-related goal of reducing obesity-related disease. Yet bariatric surgery is often advertised as a means to improve lifestyle and sex drive. In addition, it is often combined with plastic surgeries that have solely aesthetic rationales (Edmonds 2013). This sequence of operations can pose significant health risks and may require multiple corrective surgeries. Even if procedures with aesthetic aims sometimes enhance body capital, whether they *should* be used for this purpose raises different questions. For example, cosmetic breast implants require lifelong expenses for replacements and breast MRIs (Zuckerman 2010). Thus investments in body capital carry both economic and health risks, which may have unfavorable risk-benefit ratios over time—even if they yield perceived short-term gains in body capital.

The body capital concept also highlights new pressures confronting the aging body. The growth of delayed marriage, divorce, and women's participation in the workforce means that bodies are valued in both labor and sexual fields for longer periods of the life cycle. Although youth is often portrayed as extending into the thirties and forties (sometimes controversially), the risks of aging are understood to begin at an earlier age. New aging norms posit aging not as a passage through social roles, nor again as inevitable bodily decline, but as a lifelong project requiring management. Health, sexual, and beauty techniques—such as the use of Viagra, postmenopausal hormones, sexual aids, diets, plastic surgery, and psychotherapies—are offered as means to pursue "successful aging" or "sexual fitness" (Katz and Marshall 2003). For women, these norms are often "aestheticized" in that they focus on the technical management of attractiveness (Edmonds 2014). In this trajectory of aging, body capital becomes a more salient aspect for a person throughout the life course. It requires management that can carry risks to health or psychological well-being.

CONCLUSION: THINKING THROUGH
FAT WITH BODY CAPITAL

We have discussed some of the social conditions underlying the valuing of appearance. In late consumer capitalism, body capital becomes a salient and fungible aspect of the person in a widening range of social circumstances, such as labor, sex, health, and leisure—fields that, we have argued, are overlapping. In some fields, transactional sex is becoming normalized, and more labor fields involve the commodification of the body. Yet body capital is not a stable asset inherent to the person (as often implied in economic accounts). Instead, appearance is converted to body capital when specific social conditions enable or mandate it. As the case of women's body capital in the VIP party scene suggests, the exchange value of attractiveness is often appropriated by those who dominate the field.

Body capital is a useful concept for broadening discussion of fat bodies beyond a narrow focus on health. The public health message to "lose (bad) fat" can converge with—or amplify—pressures to manage body shape in sexual and labor fields. However, tensions also exist between the way fat is valued in public health and how it is valued elsewhere—a fact that has important health implications. An obvious irony in current American discourse around body shape is that a gap exists between aesthetic ideals and health norms, with both values becoming increasingly distant from the average population weight. These gaps have been blamed for disordered eating and fat shaming and perhaps indicate a need for rethinking the paradigm of body-weight management in public health.

We hope this discussion—along with other chapters in the book—stimulates new approaches to an ecology of fat in which not only the biological or lifestyle factors that make people fat but also the symbolic and economic environments that make fat "good" or "bad" are taken into account. In addition to being valued in medical discourse for its health consequences, fat is aesthetically and materially valued in the porous fields of leisure, labor, and sex. The "war on fat" is harmed by a narrow focus on fat as the target of interventions, instead of a broader approach that also considers the relationships people have to their environments and to each other.

NOTES

1. Catherine Hakim (2010) presents a typology of six attributes of erotic capital: beauty, sexual appeal, liveliness, social skills and charm, social presentation (style and dress), and sexuality (competencies, imagination, etc.). In their study of female sex workers in China, Ding and Ho (2012) name four "currencies" of sexual capital: bodily beauty, sexual practices and skills, performance (entertainment and gender performance), and sexual and emotional sophistication. While such classificatory schemas are somewhat arbitrary, they suggest that perceptions of attractiveness involve a combination of inherited and learned qualities.

2. See Bourdieu (1993) for a discussion of similar polarization in the field of cultural production.

CHAPTER THREE

Fat and Too Fat

Risk and Protection for Obesity Stigma in Three Countries

EILEEN P. ANDERSON-FYE, STEPHANIE M. MCCLURE, MAUREEN FLORIANO,

ARUNDHATI BHARATI, YUNZHU CHEN, AND CARYL JAMES

In an era of accelerating global obesity rates and increasing attention to the health risks of being overweight or obese, the question "How fat is too fat?" can begin to sound rhetorical. Obesity rates have more than doubled since 1980 (WHO 2015c). The World Health Organization has dubbed it a global "epidemic" (WHO 2015a) for more than a decade, and in 2014 its global economic impact was estimated to be $2 trillion (Dobbs and Sawers 2014), an amount comparable to the financial effects of tobacco or war and violence and 40 percent more than alcoholism worldwide.

It is perhaps little wonder, then, that while society experiences the associated health crises, negative social interpretation and judgment globally regarding obesity and overweight also have been growing (Puhl et al. 2015; Andreyeva, Puhl, and Brownell 2008; Brewis 2010; Sobal 1991). This stigma has extended to areas where fat previously had been considered positively as a sign of prestige and sometimes economic success (Brewis 2011). But although opinions abound regarding the reasons for the proliferation of such attitudes worldwide—for example, the spread of "Western" (i.e., North American) dietary and physical activity practices and media—little is known about the predictors and processes of the rise of fat stigma in the developing world (Brewis and Wutich 2012). Even less is understood about individuals' experiences and meaning making around shifts in body size, body-size ideals, and fat stigma (Anderson-Fye 2012). As a result, researchers to date have been able to offer limited insight regarding why rates of obesity and stigma are not strictly linear.

It is known that a "tipping point" of economic prosperity exists where a population with a previously high percentage of underweight population suffering undernutrition sees an increased rate of overweight individuals. Among low- and middle-income countries, for example, weight predicts wealth and vice versa. Among middle-income countries, some inversion of the relationship is noted, and among industrialized nations, greater weight is increasingly tied to relative poverty (Hruschka 2012). This tipping point can also signal the moment when the idea of fatness as an undesirable personal and social characteristic begins to become more common. Yet the individual pace, process, and practice of internalization of this fat stigma are likely highly varied.

Once present, however, the effects of stigma itself appear to be far more consistent. In the United States, fat stigma explains the relationship between high body mass and lower professional and educational access; reduced pay; lack of access to quality health-care service; susceptibility to firing, bullying, teasing, and romantic rejection; and high rates of depression and low self-esteem (Puhl and Brownell 2003). Similar trends can be seen in developing countries. In the wake of modernization, wage-earning opportunities in tourism are afforded preferentially to young, slim, comely females (Becker 2003; Anderson-Fye 2004; Becker 2004; Edmonds 2010; Katzman et al. 2004). In many parts of the world, market economics and globalization processes seem to have driven the overturn of the centuries-old association between body mass and prosperity (see Hruschka, this volume). Some simply argue that as resource access and prosperity become increasingly aligned with one body size, stigma against the "opposing" body size rises.

Human behavior, embedded as it is in cultural and historical processes and social structures, is not so straightforward. To date, the mechanisms by which wealth, weight, and fat stigma interrelate have not been well understood (cf. Brewis and Wutich 2014). Similarly, few explanations have been offered regarding the variation in, process of, and individual engagement with the proliferation of fat stigma and the relation of fat stigma to other important components of body image. Given the enormous economic, physical, and emotional costs of both obesity and stigma, this dearth of information and insight is particularly striking (Yach, Stuckler, and Brownell 2006) and worrisome.

Understanding relationships among body ideals, upward mobility, and obesity stigma has the potential to inform theoretical cultural anthropology, particularly in terms of modifications in symbolic body capital in the context of sociocultural change. Additionally, enhancing our knowledge of how these dynamics instantiate and gain currency in individuals' lives carries the enormous potential to enhance the effectiveness of interventions in global health and well-being. The work presented here investigates these multiple simultaneous meanings of obesity and stigma among young adults by drawing on research in three countries: Belize, Jamaica, and Nepal. This work can inform knowledge of how obesity stigma develops as well as what is "at stake" in different contexts regarding the meaning of body sizes and shapes.

Body and Meaning

Rates of obesity have more than doubled worldwide over the past thirty-five years (WHO 2015c). Though excess weight has traditionally been associated with resource abundance, much of the recent rise in obesity has occurred among the poor of developing and developed nations. An "obesity paradox" has emerged in which undernutrition and overnutrition coexist in both developing nations and within complex developed nations as related to structural inequality (WHO 2015b). Though common neoliberal framings of obesity in the United States and other developed nations tend to characterize the worldwide trend toward increasing body size and its differential manifestation in populations as simple matters of preference or lifestyle choice, such a simplistic and individualistic explanation is ethnocentric as well as inaccurate.

The rise in obesity prevalence is a result of a complex web of structure and agency, genetics and environment, beliefs and behaviors (Brewis 2011; Keith et al. 2006). Issues of food access (cost and quality), built environment opportunities and constraints (neighborhood recreational capacity and safety), heredity, and culture all play a role (NIH 2014). Now that obese body mass index (BMI) has evolved from a descriptive "condition" to a medically managed "disease," as it has recently in the United States (e.g., Field, Camargo and Ogino 2014), individualization and "medicalization" of obesity are further pronounced.

As rates and proportions of overweight shift, so do the meanings attached to various body shapes and sizes (Anderson-Fye 2012). Because obesity is increasingly associated with "have not" status marked as uniformly "sick," stigma against obesity appears to be increasing (Brewis and Wutich 2014; Brewis, Hruschka, and Wutich 2011). Obesity *stigma* can circumscribe life chances through negatively affecting employment, job advancement, marriage prospects, the number and quality of personal relationships, and emotional and psychological health (Brownell et al. 2005). However, stigmatized meanings of obesity are culturally and historically specific. For example, there are data suggesting that the relationship between obesity and health status may be variable (e.g., Sundborn et al. 2008), and historically and cross-culturally large bodies have held the status of "health" (Anderson-Fye 2012; Popenoe 2004). Obese bodies are likely to have multiple simultaneous meanings in contexts that are undergoing rapid sociocultural change (Anderson-Fye 2011, 2012; Brewis 2011).

Obesity + Poverty = Stigma?

The paired rise in obesity prevalence and obesity stigma initially can seem contradictory—at first glance it would seem that gain in one would decrease the other. Understanding this apparent contradiction relies, at least in part, on the ways that improvement in economic well-being affect body size. Access to foods (access includes issues of storage and cost per serving) of high nutritional quality is positively correlated with socioeconomic status in many developed and developing countries (Darmon and Drewnowski 2008). The reliance among poorer populations on low cost, calorie-dense, nutritionally meager foods contributes to obesity rates being highest among those who are the least well off.

We then might suspect that presence and strength of obesity stigma are also associated with socioeconomic status, with the stigma being strongest among those who are affluent and least strong in communities in which poverty is endemic and opportunities for upward mobility are perceived as limited. There is evidence to support such a relationship (Brownell et al. 2005). However, socioeconomic status does not predict obesity stigma perfectly. This is in part because there is no universal human body aesthetic. Cultural notions of a "good body" are influenced by history, gender norms, general health conditions, and the nature of work, among other factors (Anderson-Fye 2011; McClure, Poole, and Anderson-Fye 2012; Edmonds 2012). Among the Taureg of North Africa, for example, female fatness used to symbolize wealth, but as younger generations are shifting from a pastoral to an agricultural lifestyle, a preference for more lean and nimble female bodies capable of working the land has emerged (Rasmussen 2010). In contrast, in local contexts with high HIV rates and limited access to medication, a lean, spare appearance is indicative of illness, not affluence (Puoane, Tsolekile, and Steyn 2010).

The economic inequality that is an inextricable aspect of complex state cultures in which most humans live also creates economies of sex. These economies construct bodies as objects of trade and accompanying sets of aesthetics that assign differential value to those bodies (see Edmonds and Mears, this volume). Both "good bodies" and stigmatized ones, then, are culturally produced,

Table 3.I. Country demographic variation in 2012 (time of data collection).

	Belize	Jamaica	Nepal
World Bank income classification	Lower middle	Upper middle	Low
Overweight/obesity global rank	Mid-low	Mid	Very low
World region	Central America/ Caribbean	Caribbean	Central Asia
University sampled	University of Belize	University of the West Indies	Tribuvhan University

local instantiations of multiple local and extralocal determinants (Anderson-Fye 2012; Becker, this volume; Casper, this volume; McClure, this volume; Taylor, this volume; Trainer, this volume).

THE STUDY

The findings presented here come from a pilot study of ethnographic investigation of fat stigma in three countries (NSF-BCS1244944). Teams of graduate, undergraduate, and faculty researchers conducted mixed-methods data collection in university and community sites in Belize, Jamaica, and Nepal, primarily during the summer of 2012. Each of these pilot sites was chosen for its unusual historical record of body-image data as well as prior ethnographic knowledge and relationships. Moreover, the countries represented a diversity of wealth classifications, obesity rates, and culture areas, allowing us to both dive deep and learn about crosscutting variation (see table 3.1).

Belize was noted to be unusually resistant to the global spread of eating disorders in the late 1990s (Anderson-Fye 2004; Anderson-Fye and Lin 2009). The same research also found a remarkable range of female bodies considered beautiful. Jamaica had been written about as "fat loving" (Sobo 1993), yet eating disorders and other body-image concerns were starting to appear (James 2012). Nepal was notable for spiritually mediated beliefs about body that would lead toward minimal attention being paid to any body size (Desjarlais 1992). However, earlier work by our team and anecdotes by established fieldworkers provided the suggestion that body size may matter in important and unexpected ways where there is slippage between instrumental and ornamental concerns in some contexts (see Bharati and Anderson-Fye n.d.).[1] Taken together, these diverse field sites allowed us nuanced comparative data that suggested crosscutting themes (e.g., the centrality of gender in every field site) and area-specific variations (e.g., within-gender variations in ideals and satisfaction by site).

The overall study's goals were multiple and multifaceted. At a fundamental level, the work sought to validate and explore ethnographically the concept of "fat stigma," including in places previously conceived as not having such concerns. We wanted to understand how attitudes toward obesity operated at social and individual levels. This effort involved assessing perception and meaning of local body ideals among young, upwardly mobile females and males. At the same time, it was important to establish the existence and meaning of antifat social norms (if any). We wanted to capture participants' perceptions of the social consequences of violating antifat norms (where such norms exist).

The study also sought to determine whether and to what degree symbolic body capital and the desire for upward mobility mediated the relationship between antifat social norms and internalized fat stigma for individual meaning making and behavioral choices.

Research Design and Methods

The results discussed in this chapter—focusing on nuanced meaning-centered data—are based on data drawn from several of the mixed methods in the larger study employed in all sites: qualitative survey responses, semistructured and open-ended interviews, and participant observation. Qualitative survey questions were both adapted from prior research and generated uniquely for this exploratory study based on the literature to date. Semistructured interviews contained questions that were asked in each site (e.g., probing for body ideals) as well as site-specific questions based on prior findings (e.g., how the tourism industry affects body ideals in Belize). Open-ended interviews followed the participants' line of discussion. Participant observation was carefully crafted to include not only college campuses and surrounding areas where youth spent time but also other specific locations where attention to bodies might come to the fore, such as gyms, dining halls, and public areas used for outdoor exercise. Thus all of the methods were designed to collect data that would be comparative as well as explore site specificity.

The sample targeted young adults aged eighteen to thirty for a range of

Table 3.2. Sample size by country and instrument.

	Belize (n)	Jamaica (n)	Nepal (n)
Survey	19	19	122
Interview (college:community)	43 (19:24)	36 (8:28)	39 (20:19)

salient reasons. Purposive sampling included university students from any socioeconomic or regional background and similar-aged nonstudent partici-pants. Undergraduates from the largest public university in each country were chosen because they are an upwardly mobile population across national and regional contexts. They form a local and global population that is by defini-tion in profound social transition since a primary aim of higher education is to enable individual socioeconomic advancement. These youth are at a key time in each context for engagement with markets of mate selection and employment, both of which increase salience of body ideals (see Hruschka, this volume). Developmentally, youth are primed to engage global media, technology, and messages (Anderson-Fye and Floersch 2009), factors convincingly proven to affect body image and eating behaviors (Becker, Gilman, and Burwell 2002).

Same-aged peers who do not attend university also may engage social body capital as a tool of socioeconomic advancement. But to the extent that their college-gained knowledge and skills have market value, individuals who attend or graduate from college may have more opportunities to employ social body capital to their advantage. In addition, they may have greater choices about whether and how to do so. Both groups (enrolled and not enrolled in college) were included in the sample to examine differences, if any. Gender was bal-anced in all sites with nearly half enrollment for each gender. See table 3.2 for the sample distribution.

Surveys were conducted online in Belize and Jamaica and with pen and pen-cil in Nepal. Handwritten qualitative answers were transcribed and included in the qualitative database. The majority of the interviews were audiotaped and transcribed; the remainder were recorded with detailed notes. Qualitative sur-vey data were entered into Atlas.ti, as were interview data. The research team created a codebook for thematic analysis that included theoretically driven and emergent themes (Bernard and Gravlee 2014) as well as specific analysis for discrepant data (Anderson-Fye 2004). At least two research assistants and the PI confirmed the codes with high inter-rater agreement; at least two other research assistants conducted spot checks. The entire research team examined the few coding discrepancies that emerged until consensus was reached. At least one field worker from the specific site and one researcher not at that site were included for each country of data with the aim to maximize validity and mitigate assumptions and blind spots in data analysis. All research was approved by the Case Western Reserve University IRB as well as ethics review in each specific country.

SUMMARY OBESITY STIGMA FINDINGS ACROSS COUNTRIES

Body Attitudes

Fat stigma was present in all three countries, particularly among upwardly mobile subpopulations. All three countries also held a distinction between "fat" and "too fat"; in other words, a certain amount of fatness was considered acceptable, or even desirable, depending on the context in which a person's body size was being regarded. The amount and distribution of acceptable or desirable fat differed among countries, regions, and genders. Those in the "too fat" category were generally considered socially less desirable. They were also seen as potentially less employable if their fatness was perceived to impede their mobility (Nepal, Jamaica) or their ability to make an attractive presentation (Belize, Jamaica). Generally speaking, the presence and size of a "belly roll," or excess midsection flesh, indexed categorization as "too fat" in all three countries. Also, there was in all three countries some expectation that female bodies were expected to be fatter than male bodies due to physiology, gendered lifestyle, and aesthetics.

The meaning of the term *fat* was also nuanced in each setting. Across the three countries, both genders, and college enrollment or not, *fat* appeared in narratives as both a descriptive and evaluative term. Sometimes fat was discussed in each setting as a relatively neutral descriptor of someone that could later prove to have positive or negative attributes. Sometimes it was used as a derogatory judgment or slander, and sometimes—if it was the right kind of fat such as an hourglass-shaped woman dancing well in a Jamaican or Belizean context—it was used as a positive compliment. There was strong evidence across all the settings in light of their historical records that the valence of the word *fat* was increasingly evaluative and negative.

Intriguing though the similarities between these countries are, their differences are equally striking. As noted earlier, the boundary between accept-ably fat and too fat varies between countries. Jamaican and Belizean partici-pants were likely to describe an ideal female body as having a small waist and fuller hips and thighs—to focus on shape as much or more than size (e.g., Anderson-Fye 2004). However, the emphasis on being slender and shapely was greater in the Belizean college student data than in the Jamaican, especially in regions of the country in which interaction with tourists from North America and Europe was common. Jamaicans disparaged females being either too fat or too thin, but the range of acceptable size between these two extremes, espe-cially if one's shape was pleasing, was broad. Few Nepalese mentioned body shape in their characterization of an ideal body; height, rather, was the second most important physical characteristic after size/weight. Moreover, the range of acceptable variation in body size appears to be much narrower in Nepal than in Jamaica or Belize; categorization as acceptably fat seems to apply primarily to rural men, for whom bigger bodies provide an advantage in terms of physical labor capacity.

Instrumentality, Gender, and Body-Size Ideals

With respect to bodies and labor, concerns with male fatness were associated with physical prowess in all three countries. Though the capacity to perform manual labor was not part of the college students' present or planned lives, there was a consistently expressed interest in performing fitness—in being able to exert oneself in sports or during working out without distress. Male and female participants in Belize and Jamaica expressed preference for visibly mus-cular male bodies, as did Nepali males. However, the image referenced with respect to this visual representation of performance capacity varied by coun-try. In Belize, the dominant desired image reported in these data echoed US male body aesthetics of muscle bulk and definition. In Jamaica, the commonly desired male body was not reported as bulky or muscle bound but featured a well-defined chest and upper arms. Nepali men reported looking to Bollywood for ideals and favored a lithe, slender look.

Though men's appearance was more tied to instrumentality than women's in all three countries, significant variation existed. Though the body ideal for Jamaican males was lean and muscular, some very slender male Jamaican study participants spoke of being "happy the way God made me" and having little interest in cultivating a more "cut" appearance. The desire for males to appear fit (in addition to being height/weight proportionate) was expressed consistently among urban Nepalese. A large proportion of Belizean males in a beachside tourist area endorsed the ideal of a "buff" and "cut" appearance, though there was variation. Interestingly, several Belizean females stated a preference for fat men because they associated a rounder, softer appearance with kindness, faithfulness, better fathering skills, and less potential to inflict serious physical harm during domestic disputes. Overall, in fact, females were much less concerned with male muscularity than males in all three countries. On average, across all the sites, women expressed more concern about how they would be treated and the character of a man as more important than body ideals in mate selection.

As the examples indicate, gender was a major variable in conceptions of weight, proportionality, and the ideal body in all three national samples. Overall, appearance norms were applied to women more consistently and rigorously than to men in this sample, though of course there were exceptions as in other parts of the world (e.g., Anderson-Fye 2012). For example, participants frequently noted that men exercised "for themselves" rather than as part of a desire to be looked at, to conform to others' ideas of how they should look, or both, whereas women tended to report far greater concern with others' perceptions. At the same time, the status of women's bodies as objects of culture does not strictly prescribe what is considered an attractive female body. Aesthetics are functions of context and power relations, and in any complex developing or developed state culture, aesthetics are likely to vary because of the multiple factors that inform that context and influence the expression and experience of power. Embodied maleness is distinct in its relative subjectivity across sites. For example, in Nepal, a collectivist developing country where caste and class both matter, variation in what is considered the "right" body for men appeared to be largely a function of work environment (mountain versus valley) and status (poor versus well off). In Jamaica, a "Western" developing country, many college-enrolled and community participants reported that for men, having money was more important than size or weight in terms of attracting women.

There is, then, both commonality and diversity in perceptions of desirable and undesirable bodily presentation between and within the three countries we studied. Setting aside the similarities for the moment and focusing on the differences, those noted between countries were perhaps not surprising. However, our findings of multiple and sometimes conflicting notions within a country of what marked the breach into "too fat" and what circumstances mitigated against such a designation were both important and intriguing. These mitigating circumstances included gender and environment as well as level of education and socioeconomic status. They are described in more detail in the following section.

RISK AND PROTECTIVE FACTORS FOR FAT STIGMA

Across each of the sites, we noticed themes that appeared to increase risk for stigma against obesity and others that produced protection against it. Although each of the sites had these categories we are calling "Risk" and "Protection," the content of the categories varied by context (see table 3.3). Categories are discussed by country in order by salience. Salience was determined by the quantity and quality of data produced around each theme in this sample.

Belize

Fat stigma today has the potential to be more prevalent in Belize than it might have been in earlier eras. Since gaining its independence in 1981, Belize has experienced rapid cultural and social change. A dramatic increase in tourism and the growing prevalence of US television programming have contributed significantly to evolving ideals regarding body size and shape. Some of the most popular US film and television stars, for example, are exceptionally thin or at the very least not overweight. As one of the study participants observed, "Now you have that figure the influence from America is really hitting here now. At

Table 3.3. Summary of fat stigma risk and protection themes by country.

	Belize	Jamaica	Nepal
Risk	Tourism and media; upward mobility;* moral judgment	Size and social rejection; male gender	Moral judgment; urban navigation; media
Protection	Multiculturalism; self-presentation; male gender	Shape and texture; female gender	Belief/behavior incongruity; instrumental capability (especially rural); family and marriage

*Upward mobility is operationalized here by endorsement of "wanting a better life" than one grew up with or has now.

first any body size was accepted, you could go into the pageants being any size, height, tall, short, any size. Now you have to be skinny to enter a pageant. Now when you do photo shoots they only show images of petite girls. It's taking over; it's no longer about being comfortable in your own skin." This participant's observations were consistent with other narrative and participant-observation data as well as historical data (e.g., Anderson-Fye 2004; Wilk 1995).

RISK FACTORS

Risk Theme: Tourism and Transnational
Media Influences on Ideals

The notion of a personal, individualized standard for one's appearance seemed to be growing far more uncommon than it had been in the past—regardless of age or economic status. Moreover, individuals frequently criticized others for what they saw as excessive size or weight. Not only did people internalize the new transnational standards with direct attribution to them, but they also recognized the strength of these expectations in forming others' opinions of them. When asked about the benefits of a body that matched the ideal, one female student study participant replied, "Well first of all you have more advantage, accepted more by society. You fit in with everyone. No one looks at you, talks about you. They want to be your friend and are not ashamed to be around you or socializing with you. If you have the ideal body you're also healthy, it's a plus." Societal acceptance and health were frequently mentioned. In a context where the "society" and members of that society increasingly included North American influences due to tourism and the industries that support it, these powerful norms took on increased import and have been doing so for over three decades (cf. Anderson-Fye 2004; Wilk 1995).

Conversely, those interviewed noted that being overweight increased the likelihood of ridicule or teasing. Worse, those with larger bodies also faced negative assumptions about their character or discipline. In one interview a participant explained that "here in Belize, usually fat relates directly to being greedy." Said another, "People tend to judge you from your appearance before they even get to know you—they will say oh he's nasty, he's overweight, he's probably unhealthy." These sorts of negative comments were frequently attributed to "how things have changed here in Belize due to tourism" rather than being uniquely Belizean. Television, the Internet, other media, tourists, tourism-related industries, and return migrants were credited with having an impact on body ideals and reducing the range of acceptable "healthy" and "attractive" body sizes.

Risk Theme: Employment and Upward Mobility

Body shape and size also affected some people's employment prospects. Respondents believed those who were seen as slim stood a much greater chance of winning a job—especially one in the service industry. Observed one participant:

> I've noticed that waitresses and waiters, most of them are attractive people. I guess it's just a shallow kind of thing or mindset that a lot of people are guilty of. Within jobs that you have to deal with a lot of people, employers would rather employ people who are attractive and who they think people would like to consult.

Those considered "attractive" who might become employed in the tourism industry needed to be well groomed and "not too fat." The slender shape appeared to be particularly important for women, regardless of occupation. Women, our participants explained, increased their chances to be hired if their appearance aligned closely with ideals for US females. Employment decisions for men, meanwhile, were believed to be driven more directly by perceptions of whether they can do the work the position requires.

PROTECTIVE FACTORS

Protective Theme: Multiple Body Ideals

Attitudes about body ideals were not wholly rigid or entirely consistent among respondents. This flexibility and variation appeared to stem in part from the multicultural nature of the country's population. Its residents could point to identities spanning Mayan, mestizo, Garifuna, and Creole cultures, to name a few. In part as a result of this diversity, two body ideals claimed broad acceptance for women—the US thin ideal cited previously, and the Coca-Cola curvy figure (e.g., mirroring the outlines of the traditional glass soda bottle; cf. Anderson-Fye 2004).

Asked about the Belizean ideal body, one participant said:

I think it depends on the culture. We have a variety of cultures in Belize
so it would be hard to pin point this is what's good about being a Belizean about weight because each ethnicity or culture has their own views or
beliefs.

The "culture" explanation appeared not infrequently in these data and mirrored
national identity rhetoric of the young postcolonial (1981) and multicultural
country. Another participant reported that "because of the diverse culture, you
become who you are. I think people in Belize are pretty accepting of different
body sizes." The acceptance of different body sizes and multicultural aspects of
Belizean society played an important role in combating fat stigma throughout
the country.

Protective Theme: Male Gender

Gender played a significant role in assessments of appearance and attractiveness. Some Belizeans reported a third body ideal for men (in addition to svelte
and muscular), one that viewed extra weight as a positive for romantic relationships. Observed a college student participant:

Girls like fat guys. I don't know why but I see that in my region in the
north they tend to say guys who are obese, they're more tender, caring,
cute, they're more understanding. So I think that's one of the good things
about being fat.

Added another:

Well for me some girls like chubby guys and maybe they're like more jolly
and fun. And slim guys are self-conscious I think being chubbier probably
betters the way you are. You're more of a gentle person rather than someone who is fit and who has all the attention they may be a little bit more
arrogant.

So some women reported or observed a preference for chubbier men, linking
their body size with superior character traits.
Among men, they were less forgiving of their own body ideals but also

pointed to a provider dynamic in which—similar to the dynamic in Jamaica (described below)—wallets and "good jobs" can make up for waistlines.

Protective Theme: Self-Presentation

Belizeans also appeared to link an individual's presentation to their assessment of appearance—size and shape alone would not necessarily outweigh short-comings in dress or grooming. When asked what about how bodies look is important, many responded with comments similar to the one from this participant:

> I think it's self-presentation and personality in regards to your weight. If you're overweight and have low self-esteem and are shy and don't consider yourself worth much, people will pick up on that and people will say it and it's a vicious cycle. But if you don't give a crap, people will pick up on that and not care as much so I think it's more how you present yourself in regards to your weight.

The increased opportunity to influence others' perceptions also brought additional risk. Self-care was seen by some as a moral imperative—people have a responsibility to present themselves in a positive light. Explained one participant:

> I think self-presentation is most important if you're really big and you dress nicely. For example, if you go out in the evening or if you go to work and you dress formally then that has a big part to play in how you look and how you carry yourself out—because there are slim persons who look sloppy. I think how you dress is more important than your actual size.

Self-presentation was extremely important for women and men. One partici-pant referred to it as "making the best of what God gave you. He did His part; you do yours." Indeed, observational data confirmed the care and resources that many young people put into their appearance for going to work or going out at night.

CONSENSUS AND VARIATION

Overall there appeared to be a discrepancy between personal fat stigma and societal fat stigma in Belize. Belizeans accepted many shapes and sizes, and preferences could vary with geographic location, educational level, ethnic and cultural background, age, and gender.

As noted previously, in some instances—particularly with men—people emphasized the instrumentality of a body rather than its size or shape. And presentation appeared to be a constant imperative. One student explained that presentation, not body size, illuminated character:

> In my personal opinion it would be how the person presents himself or herself because that will help you see beyond how the person looks but you accept the person for who he or she is. But it doesn't matter if the person is small or big—so the way the attire fits will help people or not give people much to talk about.

Indeed, those in tourism-heavy areas who held gym memberships reported spending up to half their per capita incomes on designer clothing to adorn themselves "just right" for special public events. Although there was agreement on the diversity of socially acceptable body sizes and shapes for both genders, individuals held themselves to exacting standards. These preliminary data suggested that those with heavy contact with tourists had the most restrictive standards for both genders.

Jamaica

Analysis of the Jamaican sample yielded six themes concerning fat stigma. These themes were balanced in their portrayal of fat stigma risk (size and social rejection; male gender, size, and opposite-sex attraction) and protection against fat stigma (shape, size, and firmness; female gender, size, and opposite-sex attraction). The remaining two themes were explanatory; they shed light on what terms like *healthy* mean in a Jamaican context and communicate an element of body aesthetics, "comfort with oneself," that has been articulated in other ethnographic studies of body image in the Caribbean (Anderson-Fye 2004).

Jamaica has been thought of as a fat-loving culture (Sobo 1993; Brewis 2011). As such, it also has been seen as particularly accepting of female overweight and obesity. The prevalence rates for female overweight and obesity seemed to support these perceptions; approximately 77 percent of Jamaican females were overweight according to pre-2010 WHO estimates (Brewis 2011). This study's findings both complicated and confirmed these prior reports.

We found a strong folk distinction among Jamaicans between being "fat" and "too fat" that varied by gender and socioeconomic status. Obesity *was* stigmatized in Jamaica, but being overweight tended to be more acceptable compared with other sites, at least for women. Within the "fat" category for women, there was also good and bad fat, namely, hourglass shapeliness versus central adiposity. Women of lower economic status faced less negativity regarding obesity. In short, neither the criteria for, process of, or effects of fat stigmatization were uniform in Jamaica.

A cultural focus on appearance (e.g., attire, grooming) and an appreciation for female curvaceousness and confident presentation militated against generalized obesity stigma. That said, the widespread popularity of entertainers such as Beyoncé and Nicki Minaj illustrated the importance of being slender in the "right" places. A young woman needed to have a "good shape" to attract the opposite sex and to achieve social advancement among upwardly mobile Jamaican females. This concern with size was also evidenced by the majority of participants in the campus and community samples who responded "Nothing" in answer to the question "What is good about being fat?"

The risk of and protection from obesity stigma in Jamaica, then, were not simple matters of assigning discerned factors to the appropriate end of a risk/protection scale. Gender, age, and socioeconomic status also mattered, as does one's overall sense of well-being and body satisfaction.

RISK FACTORS

Risk Theme: Size and Social Rejection

Jamaicans appeared to confirm the notion that, in their country, full buttocks and plump breasts were key elements of an attractive female form. These sentiments did not translate, however, to a wholesale endorsement of the concept of "the bigger the better." Jamaican participants distinguished between "fat" and "obese." Not one of the fifty-five participants from this site identified "obese" as a desirable state.

The term *fat*, meanwhile, could take on a complimentary, neutral, or derogatory connotation. Both *obese* and *fat* (when said with a derogatory tone) indexed a degree of social unacceptability. Study participants shared that an obese person might have trouble advancing professionally, making friends or attracting a romantic partner. Worse, this individual might only be allowed to sit in the front seat of a cab so as not to jeopardize additional fares and was unlikely to secure a position at one of the resorts or high end restaurants that cater to foreign tourists. The comments below, from college students age eighteen to twenty-five, were representative of the challenges of being too fat:

> You have to work that much harder to be recognized socially. Friends and people around you are influenced by attractiveness. When you try to step out and make your mark, people look at you in a negative light and think you are trying to rock the boat. They respond to your attempts with, "you should stay in your social strata and not disrupt the rest of us." You are more likely to be dismissed. People would question why you're trying to be seen and noticed if you're not a good size.

> People don't want to go out with you. You call negative attention to yourself. You get stares if you are oversized.

> I don't think it's bad so much, but it [overweight] can have health effects and is kind of creepy. You don't always find the right clothes, and your clothes don't look good when you're obese. Fat people experience some judgment and discrimination by others. The reaction to them is, "Eeww!"

These observations each described others—that their experience of obesity stigma is observed rather than felt firsthand. The impact, however, could be very influential, as Jamaicans are known to openly verbalize their views on body shapes and body size. Such open remarks seemed to have left an indelible impression as these young women were less likely to be overweight or obese than their community counterparts.

Risk Theme: Male Gender, Size, and Opposite-Sex Attraction

Although issues of weight and size for Jamaican women were rendered somewhat equivocal by considerations of curvaceousness and presentation, these subjects carried far more definitive meanings for men. Those older than thirty-five, for example, could weigh a bit more than they had earlier in life, but younger males were held to a more exacting standard by both men and women. They were expected to be lean — in particular, with regard to their waists. Most female respondents reported that they found fat men unattractive, and even men who did not possess a lean waist spoke of their stomachs in terms of a transgression of standards — albeit a transgression they did not feel an urgency to rectify. Consider the following quotations from the interviews:

> A good-looking man is more appealing [to women] than a fat man with a big belly.

> First of all, I can't see myself having sex with a fat guy, so . . . if I can't see myself having sex with him, then it not gon' work out.

> Them big ole belly and them don't care, because guys out there, where do you find a guy that is insecure about his body?

These results suggested that fat stigma was simultaneously greater and not as great for men than for women in Jamaica. It is greater in that the trim-waist criterion that left little room for acceptable variation. Thus there was less of a distinction between "fat" and "too fat" for men. Age was the primary basis for what might be termed a "waist allowance"; although a man's wealth also provided some balance to a less-than-ideal body shape or size. Specifically, some respondents observed that having ample financial resources made a man's physique less of an issue with women. Although the weight and size standards for Jamaican men appeared more stringent than for women, a "good wallet" appears able to stand in for a "good body."

PROTECTIVE FACTORS

Protective Theme: Shape, Size, and Firmness

Crucial to understanding many Jamaicans' appreciation of larger female bodies was that shape and texture are equally important — and sometimes more important — considerations than size in terms of judgments of their attractiveness. The preferred female body shape was the Coca-Cola shape: full thighs and buttocks, an ample bust, a small waist, and a flat stomach. Respondents confirmed that Jamaican females trying to gain weight do not aspire to fatness per se, but to more bountiful "boobs and butt."

Concomitantly, respondents observed that they knew women who had cut back on or completely stopped weight-loss activities for fear that they were losing too much flesh in these two critical regions. It seemed, then, that the "preference for larger female body size" was limited to a particular pattern of fat distribution. Tissue tone was also an important consideration. Larger, firm bodies were seen as very different from larger, flabby bodies. "Wagga-wagga" was a descriptive term applied to a large person whose fat moved asynchronously from the rest of her body. Fat bodies that were toned, physically coordinated, and well attired were considered attractive. One participant described how shape trumped size for her: "Oh, shape is way more important. . . . I've got shape. And that is why I don't feel too bad! [Laughs.] I'm, I'm, I look like a two-liter bottle [giggles]." Another described her appealing fuller shape:

> Yeah, yeah, yeah, yes, yes, and you get a lot of compliments about your bottom, whatever, and you know when you have on the right bra and breast is, the breasts are properly placed on the chest, yes [both laugh]. Oh yeah, yeah, yeah . . . ya get, ya get the looks and you get comments. . . . It gives you confidence to know that you're a s-e-exy fat girl!

This community participant confirmed that is possible to be a "sexy fat girl." Further, another participant described how women should not become so slender they lose their shape, especially the full shape of the hips, thighs, and buttocks:

> She'll stop, even if it's healthier to just lose the weight, she'll say, no mon, I'm not going to lose any more weight, if it means I'm going to lose weight off of my butt. It's a big part of the sex appeal here. She'll tell you. Jamaica is not a place where you'll see many breast implants, because it's not about the breast, but the hips, the thighs and the ass.

However, two male participants below reminded the researchers that the full shape had certain limits and had to move correctly.

> M1: Yeah, you can't have the wavy arms.
> M2: Or a tsunami around you. Woooo.
> M1: Yeah, we don't want that.

Size, shape, and texture combined in the Jamaican conception of female attractiveness to create an ideal that was simultaneously formulaic and flexible. Fat distribution was critical as well, so much so that size *could* become a secondary consideration to shape, but there was no strict hierarchy of importance. The importance of tone to estimation of a good body added a sense of kinesthesia to the notion of an ideal body that has been largely absent from the dominant female body ideals in the United States. Tone in Jamaica did not seem to be comparable to the value placed on female muscularity in the dominant US ideal, which emphasized muscle definition (i.e., visible muscularity)—tone in the Jamaican sense seemed to incorporate both sight and touch.

Protective Theme: Female Gender, Size, and Opposite-Sex Attraction

The aesthetic that female fleshiness was tactilely appealing to Jamaican males carried through to the second protective theme identified in the data. According to respondents, larger female bodies were visually appealing because fuller buttocks, thighs, and breasts tended to accompany a larger body size. Larger female bodies also were kinesthetically appealing because the experience of physical contact with full, soft flesh offered a distinctly satisfying sensory experience of warmth, capacity, and nurturance. An abundance of flesh—so long as not "flabby"—seemed to appeal to a sense of gendered aesthetics. Consider the following interview with two male participants:

I1: So what's this about a woman looking strong? What's the positive connotation?

M1: Big boned.

M2: I mean, the positive is that—

M1: It's a wild ride!

M2: Yes, for Jamaican men, its, its—

M1: It's a wild ride. She can go the extra mile in bed. She's warm! That warmth.

M2: For Jamaican men, it's that warmth. You asked earlier, what's the benefit of all that extra cushion and all that. A man's supposed to be tough and—

M1: And some men tend to enjoy sex with plus size women.

ɪɪ: Why?

ᴍɪ: I don't know, some say it's warmer . . .

ɪɪ: . . . I see.

ᴍ2: More to work off. No it's just that when a woman has a little fat on her, you feel a little, what word is it . . . what should I say . . . nurtured. You feel nurtured. When you play football with your brother you expect him to be tough, you don't expect to get all sentimental and mushy. Jamaican men go for ladies with a little more flesh. You feel different. You hugging up your girl she's not reminding you of playing ball with the fellahs.

Jamaican male preferences concerning female size and shape, then, may have represented a conceptualization of heterosexuality as a condition of visual and tactile contrasts reflective of a sharply dichotomized view of gender. This insight served as a reminder of the multiple realities that the body inhabits and the interaction of those realities. Body ideals reflected not only appearance and physiological function but also social and political function. The prioritization of these realities followed no universal order but was determined culturally.

If the Jamaican worldview was characterized by strong gender dichotomy and a strong sensory connection between experience and meaning, widespread intolerance of females being overweight would be illogical. Such disapproval would undermine what appear to be cultural conceptions of both the social body and the body politic (Scheper-Hughes and Lock 1987). An embrace of the lean, muscular female body ideal of the dominant US culture might offer a significant challenge to understandings about how physicality informed everyday relationships between men and women in Jamaica.

CONSENSUS AND VARIATION

The consensus in Jamaica was that female bodies should be shapely, with full buttocks, thighs, and breasts, small waists, and flat stomachs. This conception of shapely encompassed a range of body sizes from slender to overweight but did not include obese or flabby. Slenderness tended to be valued more highly among upwardly mobile young women than among women in the community at large, though body-size preference did not map precisely to socioeconomic status in the sample—that is, women in the community sample also aspired to or worked to maintain slender bodies. Jamaican females cited appearance and health as the most common reasons for watching their weight. Men were most concerned with females' attractiveness; the health risks of overweight and obesity were reasons, in the eyes of men, for women to sacrifice a degree of shapelessness.

The consensus regarding Jamaican male bodies was that they should be lean, at least until early middle age. The hallmark of a good body for younger male Jamaicans was a flat stomach. In the eyes of Jamaican females, muscle definition was less important to attractiveness than the absence of extra flesh.

Although these standards were well known and embraced, a strong sense of individual variation in body proportions also influenced opinions regarding attractiveness. This sensibility was displayed in participant references to being "healthy" and "comfortable in your own skin." Participants made a distinction between "skinny" and "healthy." One participant commented, "In my view, what you are missing: I think a man likes to see a woman who looks healthy. Not too skinny, not over weight, you know? Just healthy."

This comment and other similar observations underscored a reluctance to impose an external standard on one's body (skinniness) or risk well-being by overindulging in food (obesity). In many cases, the respondents clearly supported individual decisions to manifest their natural size and shape (of course, notions of what is "natural" are also culturally informed). That natural size and shape was indexed by a sense of comfort in one's own skin, which, according to participants, is not size-prescriptive: "'Cause, that's very . . . um . . . maybe [being a certain size] that's good for you, but then, it's all about being comfortable in your own skin."

Although the notion of Jamaican body ideals as an amalgam of cultural, scientific, and personal ways of knowing about weight and health was certainly not as straightforward and measurable as international BMI standards or standardized silhouettes, it did offer insight into how multiple body ideals might have come to exist in Jamaica.

Nepal

Fat stigma appeared prevalent in Nepal, visible through articulated beliefs as well as enacted behaviors. A majority of Nepali respondents revealed that they felt that being fat was highly negative, equating it with laziness as well as a lack of capacity for both hard physical labor and everyday exertion. On the other hand, when asked about mate selection, many of the college participants did not understand the question of what body size or shape would be desirable since the traits that made for a desirable partner had nothing to do with physical appearance. Data analysis revealed the following underlying patterns that help account for the seemingly contradictory findings in Nepal at first reading of the interviews.

RISK

Risk Theme: Character Judgments

Almost all of our respondents said that they thought fat people were lazy and did not take care of themselves. Overwhelmingly, participants viewed maintaining an appropriate weight and clean, groomed appearance as signs of health. In fact, respondents went so far as to indicate such behaviors represented morally good self-discipline and character.

Problematic aspects of the prevalence of such assumptions involved the treatment that the overweight and obese experienced. These attitudes extended to comments and behaviors. Those interviewed noted that peers often mock or make fun of fat people—even friends openly call them fat (*mote/moti*) and tease them. Although some of the teasing was ostensibly benign (see discussion below), some engaged moral critiques that impeded character based on body shape or size. For example, the same robust body that might be lauded in the rural highlands as capable of rigorous work might be critiqued in the urban environment as proof of undisciplined character.

The following quotations from urban young adults illustrate the moral connotations and the link to individual responsibility for health:

> Fat people are not devoted to their job, they are willing but their body does not support. Fat people are often sick. . . . Uneasy, always feel other people will comment on them. Negative feelings, they always think about it. People will tease fat people. . . .

> Fat people are lazy, they don't care about health. Health is a valuable property for life wanted by everyone.

Laziness and health were thought to be incompatible for those with both urban and rural backgrounds. Fatness was particularly associated with laziness in the urban environment, and thus stigmatized.

Risk Theme: Urban Navigation

Many respondents spoke about the difficulties fat people face when walking the crowded streets of the capital city, Kathmandu. Because these individuals took up more space and typically moved at a slower pace, they experienced extensive jostling and occasional glares. Said one of those interviewed: "[Fat people] can't walk or work nicely. . . . They can't run in an emergency."

Yet the challenges of perambulating paled compared to those of securing public transportation. "If people are very fat and wave for a microbus," one study participant said, "the bus will not stop." Added another, "[Fat people] can't go to crowded areas like the bus. [They] occupy two seats in the bus, [they] should buy two tickets." These concrete instrumental concerns appeared throughout the majority of the interviews in Katmandu. Although urban navigation may seem mundane, its effects were potent on attitudes toward larger bodies.

Risk Theme: Media Ideals

Study participants also reported ornamental concern about the body. Between increasing Western influences and the growth of Bollywood movies from India, Nepalese are exposed to powerful media messages regarding the desirability of muscled, trim male heroes and slim, svelte leading ladies.

Several of those interviewed cited these examples as spurs to go to the gym or start other kinds of exercise regimens—not only for health but also for aesthetic reasons. "Angelina Jolie has the perfect body," a male participant declared. "It should be an ideal for Asian girls as well." And although slender body ideals for men were endorsed by both women and men, several men cited the desire to work out solely for how they would look with increased muscularity unrelated to instrumental concerns.

In our sample, media influence on body ideals appeared to be more pronounced among data from men regarding both males and females. Perhaps because the average BMI of the female sample was relatively low (mean = 20.93), they saw themselves as more consistent with slender Bollywood heroines. Certainly among the college student females, some of the protective factors below were also working to mitigate media influence.

PROTECTION

Protective Theme: Behavior/Belief Incongruity

Some sociocultural factors mediated the weight of stigma. Even some of those who admitted that they make fun of fat people also emphasized that the teasing was all convivial and that "it is nothing serious." The teasing did not indicate a hatred of fat people, they said; rather, it seemed to be simply a social reaction to the overweight who are still relatively uncommon in Nepal (e.g., the global obesity rank is in the lowest category according to WHO 2014).

Others acknowledged the stigma associated with being overweight but also dismissed those who mocked these individuals. Said one: "[The] intellectual man does not have discrimination. People who lack knowledge will have [it.]" Such teasing, added another, is something "only the illiterate people do."

These respondents suggested that even though they may harbor negative thoughts about fat people, they would never act upon them, because that kind of uncouth, vulgar behavior was associated with the less educated classes. One student went so far as to call the discrimination against overweight people on urban buses an issue of "human rights." If people were educated, she explained, they would not charge a higher fare or refuse to carry larger passengers. College students, in particular, reported wanting to distance themselves from fat-based teasing and other behavior seen to be based in ignorance.

*Protective Factor: Familiar Structure
and Instrumental Purpose*

Although family members might openly tease one another, they would not tolerate such behavior from outsiders. The extant extended family structure and close familial relations put the overweight under an umbrella of protection by a group that accepts them based on being kin.

In addition, a larger body size could be related to an increased capacity to do manual work, like carrying large amounts. This attitude was more common from and toward those in rural areas, where larger bodies are better equipped to handle the cold climate and mountainous terrain. However, some of the remnants of this thought process lingered in the city as well in that there is allowance for variation in ideals "depending on what one's daily tasks are like." If more manual strength is needed, larger bodies are accepted.

CONSENSUS AND VARIATION

The majority of Nepali respondents equated fat with being lazy and unhealthy. In the populous urban setting of Nepal's capital, small body size was associated with nimbleness, which is essential for navigating crowded streets. Fat people were relatively uncommon and thus were conspicuous. Respondents reported that it is a commonly held belief that fat people suffered significant stress because of their visible status as outliers. In addition, participants emphasized that fat was also thought to contribute greatly to chronic diseases such as diabetes and coronary heart disease.

As noted previously, the proliferation of Western media and Bollywood movies has begun to influence Nepalis' perceptions of body ideals. The muscled male hero and lithe female lead were ubiquitous, further reinforcing the appeal of these body types—and by extension, negative perceptions of variations from it. In addition, the nation's rapid modernization has increased the number of professional office positions in urban areas, which also has raised body consciousness regarding pedestrians, public transportation, and work spaces.

Even with these broad influences on attitudes, some intracultural variation persisted. In the more urbanized area of Kathmandu Valley, for example, a fair amount of consensus existed that people prefer a slim body type. For those from mountainous or remote regions (usually populated more with people of Mongolian and Tibetan ethnicities), fat was seen as an indicator not just of wealth and food resources but also of strength, physical capability, and of the hardiness necessary to survive in a hilly, rugged environment.

The pursuit and legitimation of an ideal body was largely gendered. Although both genders in the valley expressed a preference for slim bodies, males tended to use more instrumental reasons to validate their own body ideals while ascribing ornamental ideals to women. Women asserted that men actually focused more on their own appearances; the more they looked like the toned, muscular hero, the women said the men believed, the more likely they were to attract women. But in a tertiary education environment, other individual concerns such as someone's character and "mental self-discipline" were reported overwhelmingly to be even more important than appearance in terms of friendship and mate selection.[2] Some disparities clearly existed between how people described their own attitudes toward fat and their observed behaviors. Further study of the relationship between attitudes and behaviors toward overweight individuals is needed to elaborate and expand on preliminary observations.

CONCLUSION, LIMITATIONS, AND IMPLICATIONS

Taken together, these data begin to give us nuanced clues into understanding cross-cultural attitudes regarding fat, stigma, and body ideals and how they operate regarding symbolic body capital. What is at stake in terms of upward mobility regarding choosing mates and livelihoods is especially pronounced among these samples of young adults, who are developmentally focused on these tasks.

Across all the sites, participants were keenly aware of the social benefits and consequences of matching and not matching gendered body ideals. There was preliminary support for the theory that the desire for improving one's status through marriage or employment was associated with the endorsement of internalization of stigma against obesity and behaviors to prevent becoming "too fat" for such mobility. However, there were also discrepant data based on individual circumstance or context that complicate a simple relationship, even in these exploratory data.

Notably, there were crosscutting themes across each site such as the primacy of gender and the fact that participants identified both risk and protective factors for fat stigma. Yet the way that each larger theme played out in the local context was critically important. For example, in Jamaica—in contrast to Belize and Nepal—men were at higher risk for obesity stigma than women. In Jamaica, positive and attractive versions of heavier bodies existed for women, whereas positive roles for heavier men were available in Belize and Nepal. These findings were not nearly as pronounced in the standard quantitative survey results, though they were stark in the interview and ethnographic data.

This pilot study thus joins a long history of work arguing for the importance of mixed methods in understanding body-image findings (e.g., Becker 2004; LeGrange 2004), and particularly when working cross-culturally. As LeGrange (2004) argued convincingly, even the most reliable surveys can only be interpreted cross-culturally in light of meaning-centered data. In his study, decades of reliable work on eating behavior in South Africa was reinterpreted based on narrative data that questioned reliability. In that case, South African students were showing high rates of disordered eating not in response to eating disorders such as anorexia nervosa, as the survey he was using was designed to detect, but rather in response to poverty.

In our case, the importance of data including interview and participant-observation methods allowed us to analyze which dynamics may be transnational and which are locally bound. For example, in each of these three settings, there was evidence that presence of global tourism attuned young people to global standards of body ideals. However, the salience of tourism in each site and exactly how it instantiated was variable. Although young women employed in Belizean tourism showed evidence of wanting to adhere to US standards, some Jamaican young women working in tourism would rather preserve their "Jamaicanness" in beauty standards that favored a full figure. Both were aiming for career success but in slightly different ways that are meaningful.

Although this study was limited in size and scope, it yielded intriguing data to allow us to hone our research questions and hypotheses for future work. Future work will scale up the sampling and use more precise questionnaires and interview schedules that probe both the cross-cultural dynamics and the local variations in body ideals, body capital (as per Edmonds and Mears, this volume), cultural change, and upward mobility.

In addition to theoretical, empirical, and methodological implications, this study carries meaning for public health. Global public health has long taught us that the best interventions draw on local strengths (Miller and Shinn 2005). Further, a significant concern in obesity prevention work is the potential for further stigmatization causing iatrogenic effects (MacLean et al. 2009). As obesity prevention programs proliferate around the world (e.g., WHO 2014), it is critically important to understand the local circumstances with respect to body image and related beliefs and practices, so that intended good is served in global-local partnerships without unintended harm.

Studies such as this one help us lay the groundwork for such careful practices. For example, this work is being considered in one of the study communities as the first author works with local schools on public health programming in Belize. Further, there is evidence that these obesity-related concerns do not occur in a vacuum. In Jamaica, the concern over skin bleaching was pronounced and perhaps more pressing a concern than even obesity. Moreover, dance hall culture was found to have significant impact on intersectional body preferences. In Nepal, height as a body-image concern was central. Body size was contextualized by urban and rural status. Thus, as we have learned in other situations such as those with high rates of HIV (e.g., Puoane, Tsolekile, and Steyn 2010), it is important to place related and overlapping public health concerns together in meaningful interventions. Fat stigma manifests locally in tandem with other pressing health concerns and should be considered in light of this health-related context.

NOTES

1. For example, Brandon Kohrt (personal communication, October 20, 2012),
    who has worked in Nepal for two decades, noted that body size plays a role in
    children participating in soldiering. If a child is too small for productive labor
    in the highlands, he or she is more likely to be recruited into soldiering, where
    alternate jobs exist.

2. Societal dynamics such as caste and religion were always in operation.

CHAPTER FOUR

Excess Gains and Losses

Maternal Obesity, Infant Mortality, and the Biopolitics of Blame

MONICA J. CASPER

This chapter explores the intersection of two public health "crises" in the United States: obesity and infant mortality. Obesity is typically represented as a global epidemic (WHO 2004), a "crisis" (Freedman 2011), and as "one of the most blatantly visible . . . public-health problems that threatens to overwhelm both more and less developed countries" (Torloni, Bertran, and Merialdi 2012). Infant mortality—the death of a child in the first year of life—is defined in the United States as an epidemic, though one that is often geographically localized (McClam 2007), and as "an embarrassment" (Kohm 2007). In a recent exposé, Al Jazeera (2013) targets "America's infant mortality crisis," asking why "a country that spends so much on healthcare and is believed to have one of the best neo-natal intensive care units in the world, is failing to ensure the health of its newest citizens."

Clearly, both obesity and infant mortality are seen to threaten the health and lives of people who live in the United States. Yet from a critical feminist and sociological perspective, these public health "emergencies" expose structural inequalities that belie the "imagined community" (Anderson 1983) of our ostensibly free, prosperous, and democratic nation. In this chapter, I investigate maternal obesity and infant mortality comparatively, exposing and anatomizing what I call the biopolitics of blame. I show that the twinned public health crises of "fat people" and "dead babies" collide both inside of and adjacent to pregnant women's bodies. Nathan Stormer (2000, 111) calls this site the social topography of "prenatal space" in which "the womb has become a point of articulation for society, a space where society quickens itself." With new understandings of obesity as a disease (and not merely a condition), and with maternal obesity considered a contributing cause of problems ranging from birth defects (Correa and Marcinkevage 2013, S68) to stillbirth and neonatal death (McGuire, Dyson, and Renfrew 2010), the medical management of pregnant women's weight has become a growth industry (Shaikh, Robinson, and Teoh 2009).

As a public health problem, obesity is often discussed in epidemiological terms of contagion. Obesity is said—in rather alarmist terms—to be infecting the nation, and indeed the entire world as expressed through the neologism "globesity" (Torloni, Bertran, and Merialdi 2012). Such language invokes images of giant, undulating pools of fat creeping through streets and alleys, flooding rivers and seas, crossing deserts and prairies, and eventually seeping into bodies, inflating them into icons of corpulent liability. Infant mortality, too, is sometimes discussed as if one can perhaps "catch" premature death from contact with others in a given population. Infant mortality rates are especially high among African Americans, and infant death—like poverty and crime—is depicted as "creeping outward toward the suburbs" (Rohde 2011), along with the African American middle classes.

Of course, neither obesity nor infant death is contagious in a biological sense. Thus the language of epidemic (Bashford and Hooker 2001) tells us more about social panics, the limits of epidemiology, and media representations of health than about etiology. April Herndon (2006, 129–30) offers an insightful critique of this discourse:

> Obesity is not a pathogen, not free floating, and never a virus that attacks a helpless and innocent victim. Instead, obesity is virtually always typecast as a condition brought on oneself. A war against obesity, then, cannot be a war against a faceless pathogen. . . . Obesity is a condition of human causation and therefore necessitates a war against the group of people participating in the volitional behaviors that cause it.

Thus the contemporary "war on obesity" has its gaze riveted on fat people, "people already marginalized in the United States" (2006, 139). A public health campaign (on behalf of individuals) in which people and their behaviors are seen as the source of "illness" and thus stigmatized, is ripe for proliferating infrastructures of education, surveillance, and intervention.

Infant mortality both complicates and deepens this dynamic. Here the targets of alarm and intervention are not, typically, babies themselves (unless they are "obese" babies—see Franklin 2006). Rather, pregnant women are the terrain in and through which battles against infant mortality are waged. Though infant mortality is routinely framed as an epidemic, interventions to reduce infant mortality rates are not generally population-based, nor are they global or even national. They do not tackle the structural inequalities, such as racism and poverty, which produce vulnerabilities. Rather, localized biomedical and public health interventions target individual women through disciplinary practices of preconception care, a form of prenatal health care that extends across a woman's reproductive life, beginning in pre-pregnancy (Freda, Moos, and Curtis 2006). Such biopolitical regimes position girls and women as always and already pregnant, nonpersons reduced to their reproductive functions (Casper 2010).

What the conflation of "maternal obesity" and "infant mortality" means for pregnant women, already among the most measured populations in biomedicine (Fordyce 2013; Morris 2013), is intensified surveillance and intervention. At the core of disciplinary practices such as preconception care and pregnancy weight management is the neoliberal rationale that pregnant women must become responsible for their bodies and, most essentially, for the bodies and lives of their offspring as well. Pregnant women are "encouraged" to engage in self-governance not only or even primarily for themselves but on behalf of the "life" within them. Pregnant women who "break the rules" through excessive weight gain, "noncompliance" with medical directives, and/or miscarriage, stillbirth, and neonatal/infant death are chastised, labeled, and even punished, especially if they are already marginalized by race and class (Paltrow and Flavin 2013; Casper 2014). Responsibility and blame are thus two sides of the same neoliberal coin.

In this chapter, I first offer an intellectual biography and overview of the theoretical tactics I bring to bear on this study. Next I turn to race, exploring specific ways that both maternal obesity and infant mortality are racialized in the United States, as well as intimately connected to stigmatization in and of African American lives. I link this discussion to questions of resources, practices, and governance, focusing on Memphis, Tennessee, as a geographic nexus of race, embodiment, and localized biopolitics. I then turn to the politics of quantification, showing how the alphabet soup of public health policies (e.g., BMI, IMR, MDG) represents a hegemonic register of statistical measurement. I conclude with a discussion of congruence between the "war on obesity" and the "war on women," provoking questions about problem definition and proposed solutions.

In examining the biomedical surveillance of pregnant women, I demonstrate how the pregnant body—and more precisely, the womb—is configured as a material and symbolic environment for production of new life. Or, when things go wrong, the locus of debility and death. The end effect is that infant mortality is framed as a gendered failure of modernity, a squandering of women's reproductive capital rather than a consequence of structural violence and social injustice.

CONCEPTS AND METHODS

My first book focused on the emergence of fetal surgery, linking the new specialty to the "arrival" of the fetus as a patient and the corresponding diminishment of pregnant women as persons (Casper 1998a). During research for that project, I learned about expensive, high-tech procedures unfolding in what I called "Capital Hospital" in San Francisco. I simultaneously grew aware of wide disparities in infant mortality across the Bay Area. Whereas some white fetuses — those with insured parents, for example — benefited from prenatal surgical intervention, African American babies in Oakland were dying at twice the rate of white babies. I pondered what was at stake in devoting extraordinary technical and economic resources to a handful of fragile fetuses with uncertain survival prospects while whole families and communities were being decimated by patterned losses of the next generation.

These questions, and the research itself, led me to sociological and historical studies of human reproduction (e.g., Clarke 1998), feminist women's health research (e.g., Clarke and Olesen 1999), feminist science and technology studies (e.g., Haraway 1985), and political economy of health and illness (e.g., Navarro 1993). Later, as I began to explore environmental dimensions of health (Casper 2003) and issues surrounding cervical cancer and the HPV vaccine (Casper and Carpenter 2008; Carpenter and Casper 2009), I grew increasingly compelled by frameworks of biopolitics and necropolitics as particularly useful for making sense of reproductive biomedicalization. These allowed me to move beyond classic questions about how health and disease are produced to a more elaborate set of concerns about how health and death are governed and what kinds of subjects are generated through governance. Following Foucault (2010), Mbembe (2003), and others, I address vital questions of who lives and who dies (Casper 2013a). Or rather, whom we allow to live and whom we let die through structural inequalities, racialized state violence, and institutional practices.

Deeply committed to critical studies of the body (Moore and Casper 2014), I have focused my work on documenting and interpreting the ways in which bodies—primarily but not only reproductive bodies—are potent political sites. With Lisa Jean Moore, I explored the politics of visibility, or the ways in which some bodies are invisible to surveillance and intervention whereas others are hypervisible (Casper and Moore 2009). How and why we see—and seek to intervene in—certain bodies and lives and not others is, we argued, based on established social orders and persistent stratification. We innovated the ocular ethic as a feminist ethnographic method for tracking, revealing, and analyzing bodies, even those we cannot see with the naked eye. The ocular ethic comes with a politic. That is, we reveal bodies because we want to tell certain kinds of stories and not others, reflexively indicating a clear preference for stories that challenge and seek to eradicate inequalities.

This ocular ethic is especially useful for investigating maternal obesity and infant mortality. The hypervisibility of fat bodies (Rothblum and Solovay 2009) and research centered on obesity (Brewis 2011) has proceeded hand in hand with the ascendancy of "obesity panic" (Campos et al. 2006). Conversations about obesity lend themselves to vivid articulations of responsibility, stigma, and blame. Zillah Eisenstein (n.d.) writes, "[*Obese*] is such an ugly term. It derides, and points fingers, and bespeaks a reckless disregard for the fleshy body. . . . It feels hate-filled, and othering" and is "too close to the word obscene." Marilyn Wann (2009, xiii) writes, "Calling fat people 'obese' medicalizes human diversity. . . . Far from generating sympathy for fat people, medicalization of weight fuels anti-fat prejudice and discrimination in all areas of society." And Abigail Saguy (2013, 7) states, "Given the extent to which fatness has been condemned and pathologized over the past century, it is impossible to choose a truly neutral word for fat. . . . The terms overweight and obese explicitly affirm a specific interpretation of bigger bodies as medical problems."

"Fat bodies" have become hypervisible in the United States and subject to surveillance and discrimination. In very sharp contrast, dead infants are largely invisible. We speak a great deal about infant mortality rates (IMR) and global epidemics, but not of the trauma, grief, and loss attached to them (Casper and Moore 2009). And although we frame elevated infant mortality rates as an urgent public health problem, we give little national attention to the babies themselves or their grieving mothers and families. This inconsistency is in part, I suggest, because it is largely nonwhite babies who are dying. If white families experienced infant death at the rate of African American families, the "problem" of infant mortality would likely be more visible and would warrant federal action. Alas, there is no federal initiative, such as the Sheppard-Towner Act of

1921 (Skocpol 1992), targeting maternal and infant health in the twenty-first century. Thus, although infant mortality is an "invented" social problem (Newman 1906; Armstrong 1986), the way in which it is understood to be a problem, and for whom, has shifted historically and continues to shift.

INDEXING RACIAL DISPARITIES

In 2007, *Forbes* announced "America's Most Obese Cities" (Ruiz 2007). Based on body mass index (BMI) data collected by the Centers for Disease Control and Prevention (CDC) through the Behavioral Risk Factor Surveillance System, the article stated that "we are heavier than ever," discussed economic costs of obesity, and noted that "there is no single cause of obesity, a fact that often frustrates experts, legislators—and obese people." Many cities on the list (e.g., Birmingham, San Antonio, Detroit) have high poverty rates, have high rates of fast-food consumption, and are racially diverse with significant nonwhite populations. At the top of the *Forbes* list was Memphis, Tennessee, previously named the most sedentary city (Ruiz 2007). Located in Shelby County, Memphis also experiences very high African American infant mortality rates, among the highest in the nation. Indeed, in 2002 the rate was the nation's highest, with 15 deaths per 1,000 live births, or "692 dead babies over a four-year span" (McClam 2007).

These statistics reflect a national pattern. In 2007, the overall IMR in the United States was 6.75 deaths per 1,000 live births; among African Americans, it was twice that, at 13.31 deaths (Mathews and MacDorman 2011). In Memphis, a city of 650,000 people (in 2000), African Americans made up 61.4 percent of the population (Bureau of the Census 2000). Like Detroit, another city in the *Forbes* lineup, Memphis is predominantly black. In media representations of infant mortality in Memphis (e.g., newspapers, online sources), images routinely depict "overweight" African American women, powerfully conflating maternal obesity with infant death. Often invisible in these images are the dead babies, although one story ran a poignant picture of three men burying a row of tiny caskets (Edmondson 2005).

The state of Tennessee, and the city of Memphis specifically, have responded to high infant mortality rates through education and counseling, clinical innovations such as preconception care, and community interventions such as training of Lay Health Advisors—all local strategies targeting individual pregnant women. By 2011, the infant mortality rate had dropped by fully a third, in part through "pinpointing at-risk mothers . . . and giving them intense attention, education and counseling during and after pregnancy" (Sainz 2013). This reduction in IMR translates into approximately seventy-four more babies in Tennessee annually living past their first birthdays, and it translates into pregnant women subjected to—and subjecting themselves to—increased biomedical surveillance, intervention, and behavioral modification.

As the Memphis example illustrates, race is a common variable across both maternal obesity and infant mortality. In the language of sociology, we would say that both problems are racialized, that is, they are ascribed with meanings of race and racial identities for purposes of domination (Omi and Winant 1986). As Saguy (2013, 19) argues, "To the extent that fat people are also poor minority women, discussions of irresponsible 'fatties' shore up prejudices against women of color. . . . Stated differently, fatness has become an independent (but understudied) dimension of inequality."

There is no obvious reason why African American babies die at higher rates than white babies or why African American women are more likely to be obese. Researchers have located racial disparities in both "biology" and "society," including genetics, eating habits, culture, poverty, and the material environment. Salihu and colleagues (2008), for example, studied racial differences in the relationship between maternal obesity and infant death, focusing on race as a biological category. Noting "a paucity of United States–specific, population-wide data" (1411), they used Missouri BMI data to estimate the impact of maternal obesity on neonatal mortality. Their study population included 1,405,698 black and white mother-infant pairs, having excluded fetal deaths, multiple births, and pregnancies before twenty weeks or beyond forty-four weeks.

The authors found that risks for women included chronic hypertension, preeclampsia, and eclampsia, "with the greatest risk measured among morbidly obese mothers" (Salihu et al., 1410). Further, the likelihood of neonatal death was 20 percent greater in obese as compared to non-obese women. Yet they also found that "neonates of black women had significantly elevated risks for neonatal death . . . independent of access to prenatal care" (1414). These findings led the authors to write that "because obesity is a modifiable condition . . . targeting obese black women to reduce weight in the preconception period could be a useful and reasonable primary prevention strategy to curtail the excess neonatal mortality risks in blacks" (1414).

As alarming as these conclusions may be, the study reflects longstanding assumptions about bodies, health, weight, race, and gender. Researchers presumed and sought to measure racial differences, thus a priori shaping methodology and analysis. Darlene McNaughton (2011, 186) notes that "women of colour, single mothers and women living in poverty are most often identified as posing the greatest risk to their offspring and targeted for intervention and surveillance." Herndon (2005, 139) states, "Obesity provides a useful vehicle for criticizing groups of people already marginalized in the United States." And Charlotte Biltekoff (2007, 39–40) argues, "Because obesity in the U.S. is widely believed to primarily be a problem among Blacks, Latinos, and the poor, these populations have been the main focus of the public health measures that constitute the war against obesity."

In short, lurking within findings of racialized links between maternal obesity and infant mortality are beliefs about poverty, social capital, and resources (see LaVeist 2005). Yet abstract epidemiological categories may confound the complex lived realities of gender, race, and class as they intersect in people's lives and affect health and disease (Schulz and Mullings 2006). In the United States, race and class are often conflated statistically and symbolically, such that "African American" and "poor" are proxies deployed to mean the same thing. Although African Americans are disproportionately likely to live in poverty, not all African Americans are poor, nor are the poor always or even usually black. However, poor blacks are especially targeted by state violence (see Alexander 2010 and Richie 2012).

Use of established epidemiological categories such as "race" and "sex" poses a related set of problems (Shim 2002). Although the categories themselves are based on populations (e.g., African Americans, Latinos, women), studies of racial difference tend to locate "race" and its culture-bound meanings inside of individual bodies. That is, race is understood to be a property of people's bodies. Race, gender, and class are thus framed categorically as inherent attributes of bodies and persons, erasing social structural constraints and ongoing dynamics of embodied difference. Thus stratification and structural inequalities are flattened and conflated and health problems are individualized through epidemiological research practices (Shim 2014). Although it is not necessary for such research to erase structure (see Williams 2005), the translation of findings to clinical and public health interventions replaces the aggregate with the individual as the target of racialized governance. This is the key "translation." So, for example, preconception care seeks not to eradicate hunger, poverty, racism, and violence from a community plagued by these problems, but rather to ensure that individual women receive counseling, prenatal vitamins, and weight-management training.

The simplified translation in effect erases the social. In moving from epidemiological research to clinical intervention, we may also lose sight of other possible causes of high infant mortality and obesity rates among African Americans. How, for example, are racialized state violence, the legacy of slavery, and intergenerational trauma conceptualized, if at all? How do enduring structural deficits—such as poverty, lack of access to health care, and residential segregation (Williams 2005)—shape racial disparities, and how do they reshape bodies across generations (Fausto-Sterling 2008)? Surely it is no coincidence that rates of infant death and obesity are high in the US South, with its vestiges of the plantation economy and Jim Crow–related violence.

Scholars have sought efforts to measure the effects of some of these "causal factors" on people's health and lives, for example, through epigenetic research (Kuzawa and Sweet 2009) and studying the negative health impacts of historical trauma (Gaskin, Headen, and White-Means 2005). Nevertheless we still do not understand very much about why African Americans bear the embodied burden of social inequality (Fausto-Sterling 2008; Smith 2013).

We do know that infant mortality and maternal obesity both are correlated with poverty and racism (see Bleich et al. 2010). As David and Collins (2007) and LaVeist (2000) suggest, perhaps we need to replace *race* with *racism* in our epidemiological and sociological investigations. (For an example, see Sanders-Phillips et al. 2009.) If we were to do so, our index of racial disparities would become an archive of racism and structural violence, and a poignant registry of the preventable dead.

QUANTIFYING EMBODIED EMERGENCIES

Discussions of maternal obesity and infant mortality often reflect a preoccupation with numbers and their textual representation: BMI, IMR, and the United Nations millennium development goals (MDGs) where MDG 4 is dedicated to reducing child mortality. Indeed, one can discuss obesity and premature death without ever mentioning actual people—only measurements, statistics, patterns, and other quantitative relationships. This approach has implications for how we conceptualize problems of the body and respond to them, which we might term the politics of quantification. The IMR and BMI are represented as "objective" measurements of death rates and body size, respectively, and they are relied on as meaningful "large numbers" (Desrosières 2002) in governmental practices related to health. Indeed, in classic quantitative sleight of hand or displacement of the real, the IMR and BMI come to stand in for actual persons, and it is these figures around which institutional practices and policies congeal. Yet the conceptual distanciation of the social has grave consequences.

Whereas *obesity* is a value-laden and contested term signifying individual culpability, BMI is alleged to be objective (Brewis 2011). Body mass index is calculated by dividing weight by height, and according to the CDC website, "BMI provides a reliable indicator of body fatness for most people." Yet though BMI is considered a useful measure at the population level, it pays little attention to factors such as musculature and distribution of adiposity (see Hruschka this volume). A person with BMI greater than 25 is classified as "overweight," and a person with BMI of 30 or higher is "obese." In the clinical literature on maternal obesity, BMI is used to measure relationships to conditions such as preeclampsia and gestational diabetes, as well as to maternal and neonatal/ infant death (Tennant, Rankin, and Bell 2011; Shaikh, Robinson, and Teoh 2010; Atrash et al. 2006).

Since 2003, BMI has been part of the United States standard certificate of birth, which lists the mother's height and pre-pregnancy weight among other information. These "vital statistics" have been used to track and assess the relationship between maternal BMI and pregnancy outcomes, and resulting data have been enrolled in the service of public health campaigns and clinical practices targeting maternal obesity (Osterman et al. 2013). They can also be localized and targeted at particular communities, for example on the basis of racial disparities, thus ensuring (and justifying) ongoing surveillance of pregnant women. In some feminist analyses, the BMI is understood as a technology that reflects and inscribes cultural meanings and ideologies (e.g., Gerbensky-Kerber 2011).

Elsewhere, I have described the infant mortality rate (IMR) as a portable abacus, a mobile, standardized, and shared technology that allows for global and local assessments of risk (Casper 2010, 2013b). Governments, clinicians, NGOs, and others use the rate as an aggregate measure to link infant death to both women's behavior and the health of nations. I demonstrated that in demographic and epidemiological studies of infant mortality, the phenomenon is framed not in affective terms of grief and trauma associated with loss of a child but as a sociotechnical object that performs quantitative, discursive, and cultural work (Casper and Moore 2009). For example, the IMR allows communication among stakeholders ranging from clinicians to nongovernmental organizations (NGO) while also serving as the conceptual backbone of educational initiatives in public health, including preconception care.

Yet although wrapping human experiences of death, dying, and loss inside a numeric object may authorize governance through proclaimed rational institutional responses and communication between interested parties, the IMR—like the BMI—is complicated by profound human variations in its broader social and geopolitical contexts (Casper and Simmons 2014). The IMR is always already impartial and imperfect, made workable through negotiated orders, conventions, and shared understandings (Strauss 1978; Casper 1998b). Neither messy realities nor women's bodies are easily containable—despite considerable efforts to contain and manage them. Linking maternal obesity and infant mortality necessarily invokes and relies on conceptualization of the "maternal environment"—the fleshy target of considerable intervention.

MANAGING THE MATERNAL ENVIRONMENT

An article in the *San Francisco Chronicle* by a family physician begins, "Contemporary mothers are lazy" (Schlaerth 2014). Admitting this language might sound "harsh," the author nonetheless goes on to state, "However, science doesn't lie, at least not often. A study recently was done at the Mayo Clinic, in part to see if energy expenditures have decreased over the past 45 years and whether a decrease in activity could partially explain the dramatic increase in obesity with its attendant medical maladies over this same time period. Women, and specifically mothers, were the chosen target of this study." In what can only be described as the voice of shame, Schlaerth writes of the food choices mothers make at the supermarket (encouraging others to "hook your eyes on the shopping cart of the young mother ahead of you in line") and comments negatively on the "conveniences of contemporary life" that lead to a sedentary lifestyle. Suggesting it will take "willpower" to overcome obesity, the article ends with a reference to First Lady Michelle Obama's vegetable garden.

Here we have "fat shaming" at its most visible—in a major metropolitan news outlet—cloaked in the authority of modern family medicine. But this article goes even further, zeroing in on "lazy" pregnant women and mothers. The article is consistent with the growing body of clinical and public health literature targeting pregnant women's weight gain as causing their own—and others'—obesity. This development harkens back to an earlier era, specifically the mid-twentieth century, when women were encouraged not to gain weight during pregnancy (Barker 1998). Although the bulk of the clinical and public health literature emphasizes management of obesity, several studies show that being underweight can also be harmful to mothers and their offspring (Han, Norton, and Powell 2011). Yet despite high public visibility in the United States of disordered eating, concern regarding "too-skinny" pregnant women is missing or lightly treated in mainstream cultural materials. Also conspicuously absent is any sustained conversation about healthy eating and nutrition. Women's weight is presented only as the problem to be solved.

The solution proffered is medical management of pregnant women designed to encourage "better" behaviors and thus healthier outcomes. In this respect, being "fat" is akin to being addicted to drugs, cigarettes, or alcohol, behaviors considered blameworthy that can and should be overcome (Oaks 2001). Fatness, too, is a behavioral issue to be conquered; pregnant women must "unlearn" fatness through "lifestyle intervention programmes" that include guidelines about diet, exercise, use of folic acid, and the self-monitoring of weight and health measures (Shaikh, Robinson, and Teoh 2010). And although heeding this advice is ostensibly "for her own good" (Ehrenreich and English 1978), it is principally for the benefit of the fetus: "If maternal obesity indeed increases the risk of infant death in the general population, obesity prevention should be explored as a measure to reduce infant mortality" (Chen et al. 2009, 80).

Significantly, when women are managed through biopolitical governance and subsequent individualized interventions (for example, preconception care or weight-management training), it is not, in fact, the woman who is of clinical interest. Rather, pregnant women are managed so that their wombs as containers for the developing fetus are (or are made to become) optimal environments for life (Casper 1998a). The wombs of some women—drug users, smokers, alcoholics, fat women, and poor women in general—are deemed suboptimal, dangerous, and polluted (Collins 1998b). Managing the womb thus also means purifying and cleansing the womb of its alleged toxicity.

Of course, wombs are located inside pregnant women's bodies, and so pregnant women themselves pose both barriers and opportunities. Clinicians cannot typically directly manage the womb (fetal surgeons being the rare exception), so women must be enrolled as allies in the cause of positive health outcomes and survivable fetal and infant life. In addition to being "educated" through a variety of public health campaigns, women may also be shamed, humiliated, and prosecuted (Flavin 2009; Casper 2014). The very fact that shame, which undermines health (Dahl 2013), operates as a primary mechanism to incite "healthy choices" demonstrates that the well-being of women is subsumed by the viability of the fetus.

The so-called Barker hypothesis (Barker 1997) intensified the urgency of emerging anti-obesity campaigns. Arguing that maternal nutrition (or lack thereof) could influence fetal development in ways that contribute to disease later in life, even in adulthood, Barker theorized a "thrifty phenotype" evolving in pregnant women in environments of scarcity and passed on to their off-spring. Subsequent research suggests that people who develop in more affluent environments may be more prone to obesity and other metabolic disorders. The Barker hypothesis and its offshoots have helped to position the womb as an *obesogenic environment*, that is, as an environment that can foster obesity. This term has gained considerable traction in the obesity literature, but it assumes a unique valence when applied to pregnant women, reducing the woman to her womb while extrapolating from the womb to the whole body. Thus the bodies of pregnant women—independent of and sometimes in direct contradiction to their personhood—are transformed into environments for fetal life.

Even some feminist theorists have embraced such environmental arguments, seeing them as an antidote to biological essentialism. Yet Anna Kirkland (2011, 471) offers a critical feminist response to theories supporting environmental origins of obesity, including "panicky misinformation." Stating that her aim "is to create a feminist debate over obesity policy," she writes, "the environmental argument seems structural, but it ultimately redounds to a micropolitics of food choice dominated by elite norms of consumption and movement" (464). She raises questions about state regulations that target women and their relation-ships with their children, such as removal of obese children from their parents (Murtagh and Ludwig 2011). Such regulations far more negatively affect women of color, single women, and poor women (see Roberts 1997).

Critiquing Lauren Berlant's (2007) essay on "slow death" and obesity, Kirk-land writes, "Berlant assumes the truth of a long string of empirical claims, such as that poor people have eating habits not shared by the rest of us. . . . The essay does nothing to raise our curiosity about these crucial assumptions, instead inviting us to sigh with each other (that 'we' again) at all those miserable, poor, fat people" (469). In addition to diagnosing the "hidden moralism" (476) of environmental accounts, Kirkland also chastises feminists for buying into the "time bomb theory of obesity" (rapid explosive growth), noting that "increased state surveillance means increased opportunities for detecting failure and for triggering a second-order set of rules that punishes nonresponse to the state's orders" (478). Of course, the Affordable Care Act will likely further legitimate and strengthen such surveillance alongside increased access to care (Johnson 2010; Paltrow and Flavin 2013).

Kirkland's important caution reminds feminists that embracing an approach that indisputably leads to amplified state surveillance cannot be good for women—especially marginalized women. And although she is speaking here of obesogenic arguments in general, her points are even more salient in relation to the pregnant womb framed in environmental terms. Intersections of maternal obesity with birth outcomes and infant health have proven magnets for biopolitical interventions into pregnancy. Women may well be "agents" exercising "choice" about their own bodies and their (potential) fetuses when they participate in preconception and prenatal care, but an abundance of scholarship on reproduction has shown that both "agency" and "choice" are highly structured and contingent. Part of this structuring has to do with the assignment of blame on women/mothers when outcomes are poor and credit to "successful" public health interventions when they are good (see Boero 2010). Both infant mortality and obesity may well be seen as failures of modernity, but these problems are relentlessly framed as failures of women and their always already imperfect bodies and behaviors.

THE "WAR ON OBESITY" MEETS THE "WAR ON WOMEN"

Should we be surprised that the convergence of discourse on maternal obesity with that on infant mortality is happening at precisely the same historical moment as a spate of alarming attacks on women's reproductive freedoms? The rise of prenatal obesity management and public health campaigns targeting pregnant women manifest in tandem with conservative efforts to criminalize abortion, restrict access to birth control, and eradicate funding for basic health-care services, such as Pap smears and pregnancy tests. On the surface, managing a pregnant woman's weight may seem categorically different from preventing abortion, but the logics are the same. In the United States, even in the twenty-first century, women's reproductive bodies—increasingly understood as beginning at birth and extending through menopause—are subject to government management and surveillance in increasingly intrusive ways.

In preconception care, prenatal obesity management, and attacks on women's health-care access, we see a convergence of neoliberalism, racism, misogyny, and "healthism" (Crawford 1980). The validity and objectivity of science is unchallenged even in the face of contradictory evidence about the effects of body weight, revealing the political underpinnings of public health interventions focused on pregnant women. Women—especially pregnant women—are subjected to an array of surveillance systems and interventions in the name of better health, better pregnancies, better babies, and indeed, a better nation (Collins 1998b). Women are urged under preconception care and other prenatal schemes to assume responsibility for their bodies, to assert their agency and choice in the pursuit of successful outcomes.

Yet at the same time, women's capacity to make and implement reproductive choices is eroded through legislative prohibitions. If women "fail" to secure healthy bodies and outcomes, if their embryos miscarry or their newborns die or they simply cannot lose that extra thirty pounds, they are shamed and blamed, and may be punished as well (Casper 2014). They are perceived as too fat, too addicted, too noncompliant, too poor, or too uneducated to know any better. Individual women—not families, not communities, and certainly not the state or structural factors—are made to assume responsibility for outcomes. And in a political context in which "choice" seems to matter less and less, women are wrong regardless of which choices they make.

Increased surveillance and invocation of women's responsibility, then, happen simultaneously with (and within) the structured erosion of reproductive autonomy. In practice, the responsibility to behave as a good neoliberal subject is clearly not the same as having the capacity to make decisions and act on them. Thinking through maternal obesity and infant mortality, it is worth considering how the discourse of "responsibility" both produces and masks women's lack of embodied autonomy. Responsibility may be a neoliberal virtue, but it is illusory in that many women are not, in fact, empowered to implement reproductive decisions. It is also worth considering how responsibility works in relation to gender, race, class, and other variables, for there can be no "blame" without responsibility. The blameworthy subject relies on fictions of the responsible subject. This neoliberal dyad itself does important work in reproducing social inequalities, whether we are discussing obesity (fat vs. fit subjects), infant mortality (good vs. bad women), their conjunction, or many other issues of our time. And perhaps ironically, this emphasis on responsibility and its concomitant politics of shame may ultimately impair the health of neoliberal subjects.

How might conversations about body size and infant mortality—surely of great interest to many, including pregnant women themselves—be extricated from the responsibility/blame dyad? One possibility might be to reframe the problems themselves, for "solutions" are typically congruent with problem definitions. In the obesity literature, the problem is framed as excessively fat bodies. Thus the "fix" is to reduce (in all senses of the term) these fat bodies and the supposed harm they cause to themselves and others. In the infant mortality literature, the problem is elevated infant mortality rates. Here, the fix is to reduce the rates.

But what if the "problems" to be fixed are not weights and rates? What if those problems are not the real problem? In a framework that recognizes human variation, obesity would likely not be considered among the worst public health and moral disasters of the twenty-first century. Situating biomedicalized weight management, including extreme measures such as bariatric surgery (Boero 2012), alongside interventions such as limb lengthening "treatments" for achondroplasia (Parens 2006), surgical "management" of intersex conditions (Karkazis 2008), and blepharoplasty in Asians to produce more Western-looking eyes (Holliday and Elfving-Hwang 2012) goes a long way toward showcasing the social construction of "normal" and "pathological" (Canguilhem 1991 [1978]). Framed through the lens of feminist disability studies (Casper and Talley 2007), the problem of obesity can more productively be understood as a moral, political, and biomedical register for making sense of and disciplining people on the basis of body size.

Recasting the problem of high infant mortality rates could mean, for example, focusing on women's health rather than maternal or maternal-child health as the unit of analysis and intervention. In framing women as always and already reproductive, as in prenatal regimes of preconception care and clinical frameworks of maternal-child health, the focus too easily shifts from women themselves to pregnancy outcomes and products (i.e., babies). Pregnant women, specifically their bodies and behaviors, become a means to the end of lower infant mortality rates and indeed, the health and status of the nation. This recommendation is not to suggest that maternal morbidity and mortality are not urgent issues; they are, and there are too few resources, and not always the right kind, focused on preventing women's deaths (Kvernflaten 2013). What if, instead of global (or local) governance organized around improving infant and child mortality (as in MDG 4) or maternal health (as in MDG 5), women's health or women's empowerment writ large was the target? What if women were understood to be whole people with a range of health concerns and needs, who might or might not reproduce, rather than simply containers and environments for the next generation?

Last, what would it mean to take structure—that is, the social—seriously? Regarding the juncture of maternal obesity and infant mortality, the focus should expand from women's behavior to the broader politics of food and health care, including access and quality, as well as the lived intersections of race, class, and gender. A focus on the social would highlight that interventions related to maternal obesity unfold within a sociohistorical moment in which systems of food production and distribution (and the biomedical obesity complex) profit from consumption of junk food. A focus on the social could take into account that efforts to address nutrition through public policy, specifically the rampant use of carcinogenic pesticides and genetic modification in agriculture, have largely been unsuccessful.

We would also need to understand the ways that racism—and not merely race—affects health disparities, as well as the ways that eugenic and antiblack ideologies undergird reproductive and other policies in the United States. Although the "war on women" has grave consequences for many American women, the poor, young, nonwhite, and noncitizens are especially affected. In short, a Sheppard-Towner Act for the twenty-first century cannot focus just on access to prenatal care, as in 1921, but must also attend to the structural conditions of women's lives that produce obesity and infant death.

CHAPTER FIVE

Symbolic Body Capital of an "Other" Kind

African American Females as a Bracketed Subunit in Female Body Valuation

STEPHANIE M. MCCLURE

Between me and the other world there is ever an unasked question:
unasked by some through feelings of delicacy; by others through the difficulty
of rightfully framing it. All, nevertheless, flutter round it. They approach me
in a half-hesitant sort of way, eye me curiously or compassionately, and then,
instead of saying directly, "how does it feel to be a problem," they say . . .
—W. E. B. DU BOIS, *The Souls of Black Folk*

With respect to the relationships among obesity, obesity stigma, symbolic body capital, and African American female bodies, Du Bois's famous observation might end with "How does it feel to be an exception?" If symbolic body capital is a physical presentation that is emblematic of a desired or valued status, African American female bodies present a particular kind of problem with respect to the current view of obesity as a health concern with significant social repercussions. African American females are disproportionately represented among those categorized as obese (Flegal et al. 2010; CDC 2009; NCHS 2014; Ogden et al. 2006; Roberts, King, and Greenway 2004). However, relatively little of the published literature exploring the social effects of obesity addresses whether and how the precipitous rise of overweight and obesity in this group over the past thirty years affects their symbolic body capital. Instead, studies have documented African American females' focus on style and attitude as markers of beauty rather than size or weight (Nichter 2000; Parker et al. 1995; Rubin, Fitts, and Becker 2003). In addition, social science has consistently documented relatively low rates of body dissatisfaction among African American females compared to white females (Desmond et al. 1989; Grabe and Hyde 2006; Harris 1995; Sabik, Cole, and Ward 2010). Finally, preference for larger female body size among African Americans compared to whites (Allan, Mayo, and Michel 1993; Botta 2000; Katz et al. 2004; Powell and Kahn 1995) has been documented. It therefore seems logical to conclude that fatness is generally not stigmatized among African Americans. This relative lack of stigma is presumed to limit the degree to which larger body size affects African American females' symbolic body capital. Thus the "problem" of excess African American female fatness lies in both its potential deleterious health effects and in the fact that it signals an underlying social quandary: If excess fatness has positive social meaning among African Americans, but global trends are such that upward mobility (through the job market and, for many women, the marriage market) is increasingly tied to a relatively slender body presentation (see Hruschka, this volume), African American female bodies, as objects in the US body marketplace, are bracketed—considered separately, if at all.

This bracketing extends to social science research. When scholars investigate *experiences* of obesity stigma and symbolic body capital, they almost always identify African American females as an anomalous group at the outset and exclude them from data collection (Gilligan 1993 [1982], 2011; Nichter 2000; Reischer and Koo 2004). This investigational sidelining marks racial dominants' experiences as normative and comprehensible. Nondominants' experiences—to the degree that they are inconsistent with dominants' experiences—are tacitly designated deviant and inexplicable. The effect is to equate racial distinction with cultural isolation.

African Americans are not cultural isolates. Rather, as racial nondominants their engagement with the dominant culture is virtually unavoidable. "Blackness" and "whiteness" are cultural co-creations; the meaning of one relies on the existence of the other. However, race is not a neutral social descriptor; it operates on a power gradient. Conditions shared across groups produce different responses between groups, in part because of that power gradient.

For example, a Toronto police officer's observation in 2011 that sexual harassment and assault are largely due to women's "slutty" attire led Canadian and US feminist groups to organize "slut walks" in protest. For many US white feminists, use of the term *slut* was an act of agency—reclamation of a term used to shame and disempower women. Some African American feminists held a different view. Though they endorsed the spirit and intent of the protests, they found the name "slut walks" problematic. An African American feminist blogger explained:

As a word used to shame white women who do not conform to morally conservative norms about chaste sexuality, the term very much reflects white women's specific struggles around sexuality and abuse. Although plenty of Black women have been called "slut," I believe Black women's histories are different, in that Black female sexuality has always been understood from without to be deviant, hyper, and excessive. Therefore, the word slut has not been used to discipline (shame) us into chaste moral categories, as we have largely been understood to be unable to practice "normal" and "chaste" sexuality anyway. (Crunk Feminist Collective 2011)

This example speaks powerfully to the historical construction of black and white female bodies as fundamentally different in nature, and to the power of those constructed differences to shape embodiment in the face of shared gender concerns.

Therefore, bracketing African American females when examining obesity stigma and social body capital reflects an unvoiced characterization of African American bodies as other. Valuing larger body sizes is interpreted as signaling the absence of a body proportionality aesthetic and precluding obesity stigma. This characterization ignores cross-cultural studies of body aesthetics demonstrating that group endorsement of fatness with no upper limit is rare (Brewis 2011)—it is found among traditional societies living in relative geographic isolation (Popenoe 2004). Research demonstrates that body-size norms and obesity stigma operate differently among US racial groups (particularly blacks and whites) but to date has not provided meaningful explanations for those differences. Current explanations rely on essentialist conceptualizations that are inconsistent with what is known about the structural and relational complexity of human society—as well as with the varied material and social circumstances of African American females' lives.

Though the unvoiced perception of African American female bodies as a problem troubles the form, content, and conclusions of body-image and obesity-stigma research, "How does it feel to be an exception?" is, in its own right, a powerful research question. Transformed into a query concerning body size, stigma, and the social value of bodies, it invites rigorous and nuanced investigation. Drawing on social science and humanities literature, and ethnographic data from a ten-month study of body and identity among African American adolescent girls, I argue for an anthropological exploration of the "exception" question in service of a more rigorous, nuanced account of obesity stigma and social body capital among African American females. Thus "How does it feel to be a problem?" becomes two questions: (1) what contexts inform African American females' body image, experiences of body size, and symbolic body capital; and (2) what might African American females' body narratives reveal about how those contexts operate? The answers to these questions provide important insight into social body capital among racial non-dominants and challenge the presumption that "not normative" means "not relevant to 'mainstream' consideration."

LOCATING RACIALIZED BODIES WITHIN CULTURE

A racial frame is typically used to examine differences in body image in the United States. Meaningful differences in body image exist between racial groups. Nevertheless, the common use of *race* as a proxy for *culture* limits understanding of how body image operates *among* African Americans and supports questionable assumptions about the nature of symbolic body capital among them. A concept derived to characterize between-group differences, race is an insufficient basis for broad assertions of within-group similarity. This default to categorical uniformity produces an incomplete account of African American *body culture*, particularly with regard to body size and shape (body culture is defined here as local conceptualization of the material and symbolic nature of the body). Although race cannot be divorced from other aspects of culture (e.g., gender and class), neither can it stand for or subsume the operation of other cultural systems. I argue that multiple cultural systems inform body-size norms and symbolic body capital among African American females, and that these cultural systems operate intersectionally (Collins 1998a, 2004). This intersectional operation produces a within-group variability that is not readily discerned when a single identity category is privileged.

The idea that multiple, intersecting cultural systems inform body culture — as opposed to race functioning as an undisputed "master status" (Fordham 2008) that prescribes it — challenges assertions of generalized "fat tolerance" or "fat acceptance" among African Americans. Fat acceptance and fat disparagement are observed in this group. However, their coexistence is frequently glossed over or insufficiently examined (Antin and Hunt 2013; Bass 2001; Black et al. 2006; Botta 2000; Parker et al. 1995; Stern et al. 2006). The coexistence of fat acceptance and disparagement indicates that female attractiveness is more expansive among African Americans than among whites. However, disregard of fat disparagement has reduced this more expansive view to a single, affirming assertion: "size doesn't matter." Applied to African American females, this simplistic maxim elides the tacit association of race with gender (male) and gender with race (white) in US society. This tacit association makes being the referent with respect to neither race nor gender a unique material and cultural position. This unique positioning makes it neither plausible nor likely that African American body culture would promote a singular female size aesthetic. And indeed, it has not. Rather, the "cultural protection" from majority-race body norms that ostensibly allows African American females to be less adherent to the thin ideal (Flowers, Levesque, and Fischer 2012; Greenberg and LaPorte 1996; Thompson 1994) coexists with racist, misogynist stereotypes that both eclipse and inform African American females' lived experiences (Morton 1991; Solomon 2005).

Given the complex historical, social, and political circumstances that inform their embodiment, I argue that African American females enact multiple narrative strains (i.e., variants) of body and identity, and that this multiplicity is consistent with their intersectional identities. I do not contest the substantial data supporting racial differences in body image or assert that those differences are not meaningful. Rather, I offer an alternative perspective regarding their meaning. Instead of constructing African American females as the body culture exception and bracketing their experiences and perceptions, I submit that body size and social body capital in this group constitute a unique case that offers much to our understanding of symbolic body capital. Positive body image and weight concern coexist among African American females. Fatness is accepted *and* disparaged among African Americans. Consequently, the relationship between body size and symbolic body capital may not be as straightforward as commonly imagined for *any* population.

WHAT IS IT LIKE TO BE AN EXCEPTION?

Pervasive body dissatisfaction has been documented among females throughout the developed world and is on the rise in the developing world. The construction of African American females as the rare exception—as a group largely untouched by these trends—is questionable for a few reasons. First, the explanation for consistent findings of relatively positive body image and general body satisfaction among African American females is tautological: African American females have positive body image because they are culturally protected from dominant culture body ideals; the cultural protection that fosters positive body image is a result of their African American identity. The category *is* the explanation. But categories do not explain; they describe.

Secondly, body-image and body-size (dis)satisfaction are treated as equivalent when in fact, body-size (dis)satisfaction is but one component of body image. Smith et al. (1999, 75) found that appearance orientation, defined as "cognitive-behavioral attention to appearance-related issues such as grooming and quality and style of attire," figured significantly in body image for African Americans in general and for African American females in particular.[1] African American females' appearance orientation scores were higher than those of whites of either sex or those of African American males. Body-size dissatisfaction was lower for African American females than for white females overall, but was not static: body-size dissatisfaction among African American females rose with BMI strata.[2] Some studies show no difference in body-size dissatisfaction by race among obese women (Smith et al. 1999; O'Neill 2003; Grabe and Hyde 2006). Thomas (2010) documented a high priority on attractive attire as indicative of positive body image, among low-income African American adolescent girls (80 percent of respondents) along with high rates of body dissatisfaction (73 percent).

Examination of body-image components suggests that substantial attitudinal and behavioral investment in positive self-presentation, rather than interest in being a particular size, could be the driver of African American females' positive body image. Given the importance of appearance orientation, it may be that the consistent finding of positive body image among African Americans is a proxy for a broader racial ethos: "In all circumstances and conditions, present yourself as an acceptable person." High appearance orientation scores indicate that acceptable personhood involves being well dressed and well groomed. Acceptable personhood is a public and social enterprise that is neither determined nor precluded by body size. Neglect of self-presentation because of body size or public self-denigration of one's body size violates this ethos; unshared feelings of size-related body dissatisfaction that are not reflected in appearance do not. Margaret Bass's memories of her childhood in Jim Crow Florida illustrate this point:

> I have vivid memories of treks to the "Chubby Shoppe" at Sears Roebuck or JCPenney to buy clothes for me. My mom and I, frustrated by the limited supply and "ugly" clothes for fat girls, felt none of the joy mothers and

daughters were supposed to feel on shopping sprees. "I get tired of shopping for you in these places," my mother said. "Other mothers can buy
pretty clothes for their daughters; there are no pretty clothes for fat girls."
(Bass 2001, 220)

The mother's statement does not indicate larger female body-size preference. The frustration and disappointment she voices are not an objection to her
daughter's size. Rather, they are a lament that her daughter's size is a barrier to
the imperative of being well dressed. Moreover, the mother's statement does not
engage her daughter's *feelings* about having a body for which the selection of
pretty clothes is limited. Being properly attired is the point.

Perhaps it is the conflation of public performance and private disposition
that has masked the variable manifestations and effects of body-size dissatisfaction among African American females. If "present yourself as an acceptable
person" more accurately captures the grounding ethos of African American
body culture than "positive body image," comparisons of body image between
African Americans and Euro-Americans are not "apples to apples" comparisons
in important ways.

Constructing African American female body image as an exception born
of race also privileges the notion of racially dictated body size. Morton (1991)
provides an example of this racial morphology in her analysis of two antebel-
lum American racial identities, Mammy and the Southern Lady. The Lady—
delicate, sexually pure, and devoted above all to her family—was made credible
through the construction of "an idealized servant companion with complemen-
tary moral qualities of religious piety and asexuality" but contrasting physical
attributes. Mammy was "physically strong, tough, obese, and ugly"—a foil for
the Lady's slender, delicate, ultrafeminine beauty (Morton 1991, 8–9). These
racial archetypes have contemporary relevance, Morton argues, because they
undergird understandings of race, "in effect continuing to endorse racist-sexist
mythology by presenting the old images as fact" (Morton 1991, xiv). Indeed, one
might argue that these images persist in the thin ideal that predominates among
European American women and the attribution of larger body-size preference
to African American women. What if the existence of these body-size norms
does not represent a faithful transmission of "racial culture" but a set of mutually reinforcing cultural mythologies? What if unremitting emphasis on idealized absolute differences has fostered the *image* of white womanhood as thin
and black womanhood as large and, over time, eclipsed the perception that

within-group variability in body size is normal? What if these images helped construct body size as racially driven, innate, and inevitable?

Kimberly Lau's ethnography of a Philadelphia African American women's fitness collective (Sisters in Shape) supports this theory. Lau's interview with Allison, a longtime member of the collective, demonstrates that African American women can embrace essentialist notions about race and size as truths that inform their self-perception. Allison recounts her response the first time she saw Melanie, the founder and leader of Sisters in Shape, teaching aerobics:

> When she saw Melanie, she knew it would be a good class for her to take. "She walks up and I'm like, 'Oh, I could look like her,' so I started taking her class 'cause a lot of times aerobic teachers are real tiny, and especially black women, we're thick, and lookin' at those tiny women, we're like, 'Uh, I'm not gonna look like that, you know, what's the point?'" (Lau 2011, Loc 1037)

Lau asserts, "Allison embeds herself in her performance of a collective and ideally imagined black womanhood—at once individual and plural—that exists in contraindication to white womanhood as implied by 'those tiny women'" (Lau 2011, Loc 1043). Allison elaborates, comparing the body size of Oprah Winfrey with that of Jada Pinkett-Smith. Of Winfrey, she says, "She looks healthy. She's the way she's supposed to be. It's like the way, that's like the perfect size for her" (Loc 1072). Allison says of Jada Pinkett Smith, "[She's] real petite, she had a baby and she's still, she's a small woman, she's gonna be small. . . . But I don't think they [black women] realize they don't have to look like Jada Pinkett Smith" (Loc 1061).

Allison's rhetorical separation of Pinkett Smith's body from that of black women in general arguably acts to "present old images as fact" in the way Morton discusses (Morton 1991, xiv). The variability in physical appearance that exists within any group characterized by as porous and contingent a descriptor as race has been overlain by a racial archetype that deterministically links color and size. Given her comment about the size and race of the "typical" aerobics instructor, Allison's combined remarks imply that Pinkett Smith's body size positions her more in the realm of whiteness than blackness—that racially speaking, Smith is a morphological outlier. Lau interprets identification of a "black" body type—and the naming of "thickness" as a racial characteristic—positively, as acceptance or appreciation of larger body size. However, acceptance of blackness and larger size as a natural pairing also has potential negative effects. Super-imposition of an accepted generic "thickness" on black female bodies increases the likelihood that black women who experience eating disorders will be ignored (Powers 1989), that the health implications of "thickness," a descriptor applicable to central obesity, could be glossed as "racially" normal, or that African American women and girls experience familial and social pressure to express acceptance of their size as a marker of racial authenticity (Lau 2011).

BODY CAPITAL, ATTRACTIVENESS, AND CENSURE

The perception that African American female body capital is primarily racially driven also ignores the complexity of the cultural narratives concerning female bodies that have long existed within African American communities. These narratives are shaped by the tacit reference to (male) gender inherent in race and the tacit reference to (white) race inherent in gender in the United States as well as by local culture. This means that African American female bodies are subject to processes of objectification that, although dissimilar to those experienced by women of the racial majority, cannot be glossed as universal or primarily positive and protective. This objectification includes the high value placed on gynoid *shape* (full bust, hips, and thighs) among African American heterosexuals. Also included are male practices of ridiculing the body size and bodily (i.e., sexual) practices of women who "belong" to other men as a means of entertainment and a demonstration of social power (Singh 1993; Freedman 2004; Wald 2012).

Photographic images of glamorous black females featured in twentieth-century black magazines provide important insight regarding gynoid shape as a marker of heterosexual attractiveness among African Americans. With titles like *Hue, Sepia, Our World,* and the *Negro Review* (along with the still-extant *Ebony* and *Jet*), most of these magazines had/have black publishers and all targeted black audiences. Though women with larger bodies were occasionally featured on the covers of these magazines, most of the images feature slender, albeit curvaceous, women (https://goo.gl/8YdZIJ). Given that most media of this kind *reflect* as well as *drive* standards of female attractiveness, these magazine covers challenge the idea that "larger" body size is idealized rather than simply *not excluded* from African Americans' assessments of attractiveness. Depictions of "upscale" black life in these magazines also suggest that symbolic body capital is meaningfully informed by class for this group (discussed later in this chapter).

Research comparing female body-size preference of white and black men has focused on absolute differences. However, substantial consensus exists between the two groups regarding women whose overall appearance makes them "dateable." In one study, both black and white participants selected an image of Tyra Banks from a group of eight images as representing the pinnacle of bodily attractiveness (Bissell 2002). White males placed a significantly higher value on thin female bodies than did African American males. African American respondents ranked a model who fit the clinical classification of overweight fourth among the ten images presented in the study (Bissell 2002). These findings support the notion that thinness is not a primary determinant of attractiveness among African American heterosexual males, but belie the notion that larger body size is *the* driver of female attractiveness assessment for this group.

Male preference for a smaller female waist–hip ratio (i.e., gynoid body shape; Singh 1993) differs by race. African American heterosexual males prefer a smaller waist-hip ratio (WHR) than do their white counterparts (Freedman et al. 2004). The lower body proportions that commonly attend smaller waists are full hips and thighs—in short, a curvaceous, distinctly gynoid shape. Valuing shapeliness means that a broader range of body sizes is deemed attractive than is the case when thinness is prioritized (Webb, Looby, and Fults-McMurtery 2004). This is true in other regions of the world as well (Anderson-Fye 2004). However, for reasons that likely have their roots in the strength of America's cultural investment in "blackness" and "whiteness" as distinct and unequal modes of being, this broader range of size acceptance has been misinterpreted as a "size doesn't matter" ethos.

African American male discourse about African American female bodies is more complex than that. Females can be perceived, and derided, as "too fat." The cutting humor of "Yo mama's so fat" jokes have their origins in the dozens, a game of verbal insults played primarily by African American males since the early twentieth century (Wald 2012). Female fatness was/is frequently the subject of this tradition of derisive speech play. Such play complicates the narrative of larger female body-size preference and acceptance among African Americans, as it indicates that preference for larger female body size is not without upper limit. Furthermore, the dozens' rendering of African American female bodies as objects of public sport (play requires an audience and commonly involves insults directed toward females "belonging" to one's opponent) suggests that gender norms and sexism are as significant to African American body culture as are racial norms and racism. Experiences of racism and its effects by African Americans of both genders do not militate against the existence or deleterious effects of sexism (hooks 1981; Cole and Guy-Sheftall 2003).

The dozens is not the only evidence that "the bigger the better" is likely not the maxim of African American female heterosexual attractiveness. The effects of weight teasing and censure among African Americans are largely unexplored in the social science literature. This is due to the presumption that because African American females on average have a more positive body image than white females, African American females' experiences of weight teasing produce fewer negative effects (Quick, McWilliams, and Byrd-Bredbenner 2013). Even in qualitative investigations of body perception, weight, and eating disorders (e.g., Thompson 1994), African American participants' experiences of their fatness being denigrated within their families and communities were interpreted as evidence of acculturation to majority race norms. Such focus on the putative *origins* of "weightism" in African American families provides little insight into the *effects* of such censure.

Thompson's (1994) data support this interpretation. Participants endorsed the imperative of performing acceptable personhood publicly. Censure and stigmatization, on the other hand, were borne privately. Thompson (1994) reported that many of her participants "had a deep-seated and abiding sense of having to 'go it alone in the world'" (112). Rosalee, an overweight African American woman with a binge eating disorder, exemplifies this perspective: "It is not easy for me to let people know how much I hurt. It is a matter of image, pride, and dignity. Having someone know that I hurt that bad, maybe they will know that they can hurt me" (112). The extent of this practice of not sharing wounded feelings—both as a matter of pride and for fear of attracting additional hurtful treatment—has implications for the *experience of* versus the *response to* censure and stigmatization in this group.

The size inclusiveness that is part of African American body culture does not only carry a genuine appreciation for full-figured or curvy female bodies. This body culture, and the larger US culture that informs and is informed by it, also provides the context for a number of potentially negative influences on African American female embodiment. Both cultures mask the consequences of gendered objectification for African American females by insisting that racial and gender identity are experienced hierarchically, with race perennially predominant. This fosters the expectation that for African American females, coping with the effects of *race/gender* discrimination, disparagement, or stigma is a secondary social and political concern.

The effects of these body culture "positives" and "negatives" cannot be understood as a matter of straightforward summation. They are more accurately conceptualized as the product of multiple, intersecting narrative strains—as emergent (and thus not entirely predictable) but not infinitely variable (and thus recognizable in the context of African American females' lives). These narrative strains are the basis of a relationship between body size and symbolic body capital characterized by *disagreement* about desired or valued status between individual African American females and their social contexts. Their very nonnormativity (female, but not white; black, but not male) challenges the notion of a singular standard of desire or value. And as the study findings presented below will show, the relationship between body size and symbolic body capital for African American females is necessarily contingent and contested.

NO SINGULAR IDEAL, NO SINGULAR VALUE

Sample and Methods

The data are from a ten-month ethnography of body and identity among forty-two African American adolescent girls attending high school in an affluent inner-ring suburb of a midwestern city. The sample was drawn from girls age fourteen to seventeen enrolled in the 2009–2010 academic year who self-identified as African American wholly or in part and agreed to participate.[3] The municipality has a sizable African American population—34.1 percent. Average per capita income in 2009 was $47,784; only 5.4 percent of families lived below the poverty level. Class status ranges from professional to working class, including among the African American population (Bureau of the Census, five-year estimates, 2005–2009).

Children living in the one-square-mile area of the post-industrial city that abuts the municipality are eligible to attend its schools. African Americans comprise 51 percent of the population of the adjacent city, for which the per capita income in 2009 was $16,581 (Bureau of the Census, five-year estimates, 2005–2009). Thus there was a degree of class and income diversity among the

African American students at the study school not typically found in a single community.

Data collection methods included a survey characterizing the sample with respect to demographics, family gender norms, body image, and physical activity; a focus group in which the participants constructed physical self-concept collages; two interviews; accelerometry; observation of physical education classes and school-based athletics practices; and measured height and weight. Participants constructed collages during the focus group, using images from magazines and the Internet and colored pencils in response to one or more of four questions: "How do you describe yourself physically?"; "What physical attributes do you aspire to?"; "How do you want others to see you?"; and "What do you want others to know about you?" This analysis utilizes data from the survey, the interviews, the physical-self-concept collages, and the height and weight measurements.

Results

Study findings support the presence of multiple narratives concerning body size, censure/stigma, and symbolic body capital within the sample. Participants were generally unwilling to endorse a singular physical ideal and insisted there was no standard "good" body. This non-endorsement of a single body ideal was expressed indirectly through responses to two interview questions: "Are there physical attributes of yours that you don't like?" and "Are there physical attributes that you see in others that you do not/would not desire for yourself?" Twenty-four participants named individual body parts or relatively immutable physical characteristics (e.g., upper arms, feet, height) in response to the first question.

Some participants were very reluctant to discuss undesirable physical attributes noted in others ("Weelll . . . I don't know. Uh, I don't know. 'Cause I don't, I don't like to judge people, so . . ."), even when assured that the intent of the question was not to denigrate but to express personal preference through comparison. Their responses instead routinely acknowledged individual variation ("everyone is different") and indicated a high value placed on personal preference and comfort with physical presentation ("We're both two different people, like, you have one person who's pretty but she'll have another person and they'll probably say who looks better between them? Um, nobody. Can't really compare them because they both have their own type of pretty, I guess.").

These comments are consistent with the importance of self-acceptance documented in other studies of body image among African American women
(Baturka, Hornsby, and Schorling 2000).

Despite this observed reluctance to express their appearance preferences in
terms of qualities deemed undesirable in others, fifteen participants did identify being "too big" as a physical attribute they would not want for themselves.
For the most part, participants with a BMI of 25 or lower articulated this view.
Four participants who were overweight/obese voiced a desire to lose weight but
distinguished between desire for a smaller body and a desire for "skinniness."
The relationship between size and attractiveness had both a lower and an upper
limit in these participants' aspirations. With respect to larger body-size preference, one healthy weight participant and one overweight participant expressed
desire to be larger. Larger body size tied with symbolic or abstract qualities like
"being slutty" and "having an attitude" as the next most frequently disliked/
undesired attributes (fifteen participants).

Responses to the interview questions suggested that participants' body conceptualizations were complex. They included both objectification and a separation of physical presentation from value that seemed to affect symbolic body
capital. Participants espoused no single or dominant body ideal; their statements about appearance were most consistent with the "acceptable person"
ethos theorized above. Such an ethos accounts for the participants' reluctance
to critique the physical attributes of others and for their privileging of individu-
ality in matters of attractiveness.

However, the acceptable person ethos was not the sole factor informing participants' judgments of bodily value and attractiveness. Combined analysis of
survey and interview responses identified social class as a potential relevant
factor. Of the twelve participants who named fatness or obesity as an undesired
attribute, nine (75 percent) were from homes in which the primary caregiver
held a bachelor's degree or higher, and six (50 percent) were from homes in
which the primary caregiver had a graduate or professional degree. Ten of
the twelve were district "legacies"; that is, they had family members who had
attended or were graduates of the same high school. This finding suggests that
these students came from families that have identified as middle class for at least
one generation. Hill (2002) has argued that generations in the middle class may
influence gender norms among African Americans. Most of the participants
who stated fatness was undesirable were from established middle-class families.
Class, then, along with gender and race, may affect body-size preference among

these participants. Experiences of race, class, and gender *combine* to produce symbolic body capital. And as the examples that follow will show, the power dynamics that attend each of these cultural systems may affect the symbolic capital of the participants' referent (class status) and nonreferent (nonwhite, nonmale) bodies in a variety of ways (see also Edmonds and Mears, this volume, for more on class and body capital).

GENERATING CONTINGENT CAPITAL

The aggregate demographic and interview data provide some support for my claim that multiple cultural systems inform African American females' symbolic body capital. The claim that symbolic body capital is contingent and contested for this group requires evidence that African American females engage with those cultural systems in ways that are patterned but not predetermined, and this claim is supported by the narrative analysis. The participants' narratives demonstrate how they make meaning of their lives' intersecting contexts.

I present the narratives and physical self-concept collages of three study participants—Ruth, Chloe, and Anita—as examples of this meaning making. All were district "legacies." Anita and Chloe came from traditional families with stay-at-home moms; Ruth's divorced mother was a human resource professional. All three subscribed to dominant-culture notions about the role of weight management in attaining/maintaining attractive presentation. None subscribed to the thin ideal.

The concept of control—particularly control of the female body—inheres to middle-class existence and was at issue for these young women. However, intersectionality seemed to affect the *nature* of the control and made the focus body cultivation *effort* rather than *accomplishment*. Consistent presentation and recognition as an acceptable person was as much or more of a concern as exercise or eating behaviors. This differs from the dominant-culture paradigm, which focuses on the body as a *product* of control, with closeness to the ideal being the indicator that sufficient control is being exercised. Participants' narratives also reflected concern with heterosexual attractiveness and the male gaze. Overall, participants' experiences of symbolic body capital did not seem to be primarily driven by racial body-size norms. Rather, their body capital seemed to reflect both which cultural system(s) informed the assessment of value and how participants engaged those systems.

"I'm Just Fat, Not Curvy"

Ruth's experience of her body capital was informed by familial appearance norms and peer gender norms. However, neither appeared to dominate her observations about what constituted a "good" body and how well or poorly her body conformed to those norms. Her family body norms did not map very well to "African American" female body norms. Ruth neither expressed positive body image nor endorsed larger body size. She did not advocate or aspire to thinness. Ruth's engagement with peer and family norms fostered a body narrative that reflected this ongoing negotiation. Five feet five inches tall with a BMI of 29.3, Ruth described herself as "fat" and confided that she felt like an oddity among her maternal female kin: "All the girls are like skinny and short and I'm just like tall and just . . . oddly shaped. I don't even know . . . I mean, I don't want to be like five feet, but I just don't want my height to be so awkward." Her experience of being physically unlike other females in her family informed a desire to be less conspicuous physically. At the same time, Ruth aspired to a bodily presentation that was not "skinny and short." She rejected "skinniness" as unattractive and instead wanted a "curvy" body (exemplified by the figure in the upper right of her collage, fig. 5.1). "Curvy," for Ruth, bespoke shape more than size—an "hourglass" or "Coca-Cola" shape: "So my whole thing is like . . . to be curvy? . . . Like I'm . . . I'm not curvy. I have like fat—[who] doesn't want to be curvy? I think curvy women are beautiful."

Ruth's valuation of shapeliness over thinness occurred alongside her personal body critique and the critiques of her body by others in her social world. Ruth equated being fat with being unattractive and perceived that her school peers did as well:

> But no one I've been to school with has actually ever called me ugly. I always just thought I was, because people would just look at you a certain way. . . . It's kind of like . . . people don't say it . . . well, maybe some people have called me fat. But like, whatever. But some people don't just say it to you they just look at you and you just like, you feel so self-conscious.

Ruth's sense that her bodily presentation made her an exception among the females in her family appeared to be echoed in her experiences of some school peers' assessments of her appearance. The silent nature of what Ruth perceived as her peers' derision did not appear to be mitigated by her embrace of

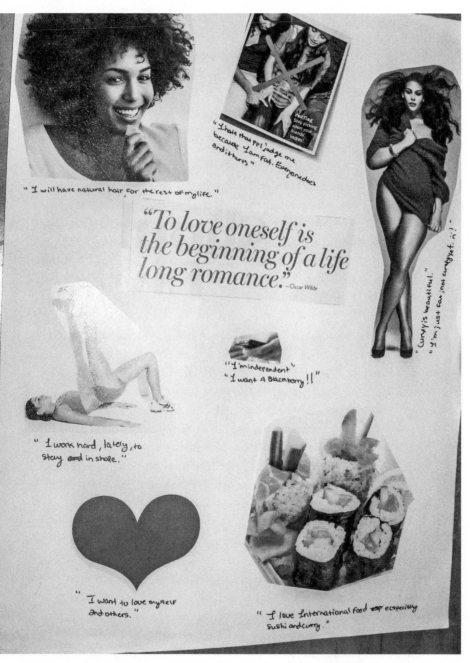

Figure 5.1. Physical self-concept collage constructed by Ruth during the focus group. Supplied by the author.

a nondominant body ideal; the two situations and their implications for Ruth's symbolic body capital coexisted. In her narrative, one context did not over-power or extinguish the other. This suggests that Ruth's symbolic body capital was *not* consistent with dominant cultural norms, was *not* absent, and was *not* readily attributable to a single aspect of cultural or personal preference (i.e., curviness).

And just as gender was a subtext in Ruth's discussion of family body norms, so too were heteronormative power relations implicit in Ruth's bodily self-assessments and her reports of her school peers' assessments. Opposite-sex attractiveness—specifically, a female's standing as an object of the male gaze—is likely what was judged during the nonverbal encounters Ruth described. In a context of heteronormativity, the male gaze carries the power of value assign-ment to its object. This assignment happens whether or not the female seeks to elicit it. In Ruth's case, the experience of having low value assigned to her appearance became part of a narrative marked by her struggle to avoid making her self-perception subject to others' judgments:

> Like, in jewelry class, we have two boys and then it's like a bunch of girls? And so, I guess one day, one of . . . I sit with one of the guys and his friend who also takes like a higher level of jewelry, he came in, and they—it was like the, I don't know, it was like, January, I don't know what, how they, I guess they just realized there was girls in the class so they started rating every—like all the girls. So they were like rating girls and like, I got a 2 and that really hurt. Like, I mean, I don't like them in any way it's just the way that they're saying, they're calling me a 2 so then, like, maybe everyone else thinks I'm a 2. Or dadadada. I try not to think about it. I try not to let it get to me. But . . . just when people say stuff like that.

Ruth tried not to let the boys' assessment "get to" her, but she did not reject it as untrue or unimportant. She eschewed thinness and advocated "curviness," but her perspectives on body size and attractiveness were not the only salient factor in her assessment of her symbolic body capital; they did not appear to mitigate the felt and experienced negative assessments of her peers. Her experi-ence as a physical exception among her female kin also affected her body capi-tal. Rarity or uniqueness can increase value in capital markets, but only if the market actors endorse the higher valuation. This did not seem to be the case with Ruth's family or peers. And it is only in the context of her family and peer relationships that an assessment of Ruth's symbolic body capital even makes sense. To assume anything about Ruth's experience of her symbolic body capital based on her racially congruent body ideal alone is to treat her racial categorization as inherent and predictive in ways that her narrative demonstrated cannot be so.

Too Skinny to Date

In her collage, Chloe addressed the question "How would you describe yourself physically?" with a trio of images of thin young women that she captioned "I think I'm too skinny and weird looking!" (fig. 5.2). Her awareness of the male gaze figured prominently in her negative assessment of her attractiveness and in her desire for others to see her as beautiful:

> Um . . . I used beautiful, because . . . or the word *beautiful* because I wanted people to see that I am? 'Cause um . . . before I like made this, like . . . you know how . . . guys usually in school want the . . . bigger girls with hips and stuff . . . and, um, to them I'm too skinny and weird looking. But then I found out later that . . . they want that now, but when they . . . [clears throat], excuse me, when they want to, uh, like settle down and get married, they look for the smaller girls, I guess. And so . . . then I'm like weelll, that's not gonna help me *now*, but . . . so I want people to say, feel like I'm beautiful like they are.

Chloe had the lowest BMI among the study participants (17.5) and seemed as acutely conscious of and uncomfortable with her body size as Ruth. When asked how she wanted others to see her, Chloe spoke first of the ways she perceived her body did not draw appreciative male gaze or attention—in her case because she lacked the "hips and stuff" that her male peers ostensibly found attractive. Like Ruth, she seemed to feel that her physical presentation fostered exclusion—if not from social acceptance in general, then from the degree of value that would render her "datable." The bodily presentation Chloe recognized as most desirable to her male peers is consistent with documented African American body norms; therefore, it would be easy to miscast the dynamic at work in Chloe's situation as purely racial. However, Chloe foregrounded her desire to be beautiful in the eyes of *male* others; she opened the discussion of her collage with this concern. Such foregrounding speaks to a female-associated experience

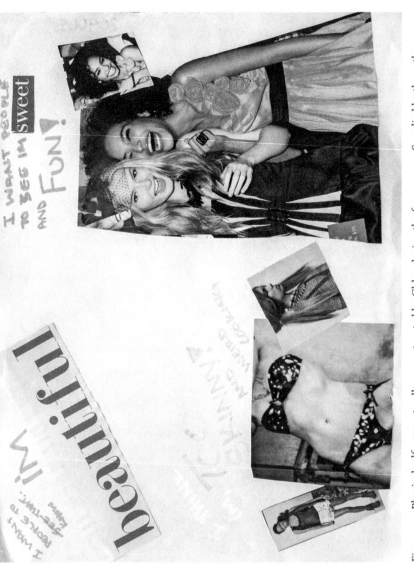

Figure 5.2. Physical self-concept collage constructed by Chloe during the focus group. Supplied by the author.

of the body that Young described as "liv(ing) her body as a thing" (2005, 39).
Her body is the vehicle of her unacceptability to the opposite sex; it is the object
that prevents others from seeing her true nature: "sweet and fun." Thus Chloe's
self-critique was a gender/race critique, not a purely racial one. This observation
is further supported by interview statements that differentiate between Chloe's
body subjectivity and her body-as-thing perspective:

> [Speaking in a very small voice] Yeah. Um . . . I guess people say that I
> could be a model, I guess, but I don't know if that's a good thing or a bad
> thing. But, um . . . I am getting clo—like, better, um—accepting my face.
> And . . . I think I'm pretty sometimes. Most of the time, I go towards look-
> ing right. Um, and then, um, I don't know, I think I have nice legs. I'm not
> sure . . . that's really weird saying, I know.

Chloe made other statements that affirmed her slender build: "I kind of like
being petite" and "Umm . . . I don't want to get, like, hmm-hmm, uh, like a
pot belly. I don't want that." Her self-approval was not full throated but was
there. And her tentative self-approval was bolstered by her enjoyment of physical activity. She grew up playing softball and joined the school dance club the
year of the study. In the context of play, her concern with the male gaze and her
perception of her body as less than acceptable diminished:

> Like, I, when I'm in gym, I usually play with the guys, because the girls
> don't do anything? And I'm sort of, kind of at that level—not there quite
> yet but they can still have fun and, with me, so it's good. Um, so yeah, I
> think it would put on the willingness of, um, athletic . . . tism [trails off,
> giggles].

Chloe's guardedly positive experience of her bodily subjectivity and her
generally negative perception of her body as object combined to produce a
nuanced race/gender/experience narrative and a symbolic body capital that
was simultaneously majority-culture consistent and majority-culture divergent.
The race/gender body norms that she perceived her opposite-sex peers to hold
diminished her object value in the immediate term. However, this experience
coexisted with an internal, perfectionist critique reminiscent of majority culture
body norms and a lived experience of pleasure and confidence in her physicality

when engaged in dance or athletics. Examined in light of her multifaceted body narrative, Chloe's body capital reads as necessarily situational and fluid, tied to no single set of norms.

"Curvy" but Well Dressed

Anita was tall, with caramel-colored skin, wide-spaced, almond-shaped eyes, and a voluminous, impressively symmetrical afro. Her BMI of 34.4 placed her in the ninety-seventh percentile for her age group. The images in Anita's collage suggested she was possessed of the non-size-dependent positive body image commonly attributed to African American females. Most of the images she chose were of African American female celebrities to whom the clinical label *obese* would apply. The words *pretty* and *beautiful* appear below three of her images (fig. 5.3). But as Anita began to interpret her collage, it became clear she endorsed the idea of being "the best dressed" (the phrase headlining her collage) — of enacting beautiful *as* a "curvy" woman rather than affirming that beauty is inherent to large size:

> Um, I chose "the best dressed" because I — like I care about fashion and stuff and like dressing well. . . . I picked those photos because like they're curvy women but like, they don't really dress frumpy, you know. Yeah, they — like they dress — like anybody, like anybody can like — if you dress well, then like, you can look good, like anybody, can look good. And like I . . . aspire to be like that. . . . I chose beautiful and pretty because that's how I try to see myself.

Anita's focus on fashion and grooming resonates with Smith et al.'s (1999) findings regarding the strong contribution of appearance orientation to body image among African American females. Smith et al. and others (O'Neill 2003; Grabe and Hyde 2006) note that high appearance orientation does not preclude body dissatisfaction. Anita's comments bear this out. When asked if there were physical attributes of hers that she did not like, Anita replied, "Like, my upper . . . like most of my body." Her collage also identified things she desired to change about her body ("curvy butt" and "nip your waist") and contained aspirational images (e.g., Beyoncé and Jennifer Hudson after weight loss). During her interview, however, Anita was critical of her body:

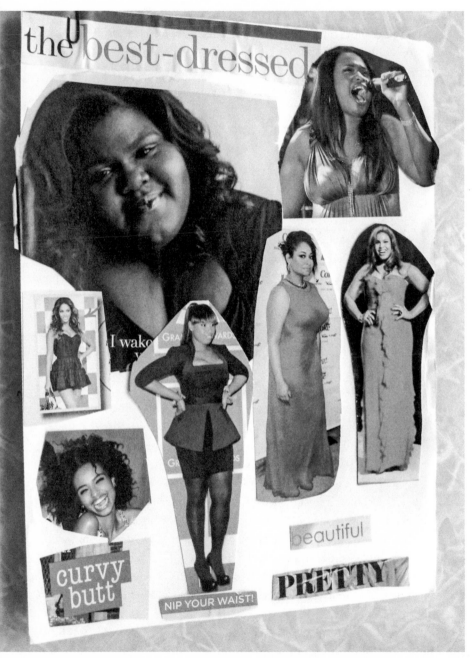

Figure 5.3. Physical self-concept collage constructed by Anita during the focus group. Supplied by the author.

I'm tall . . . and . . . I'm curvy. Well, yeah [chuckles]. Like I'm—I dunno, I have a weird body [laughs]. Like . . . 'cause I don't like have like strong curves like Beyoncé, but like I—like I have meat on me. So . . . like I've had problems with, like, I've had problems with like with my weight. [SMM: Mm-hmm.] And then like with my parents like telling me I need to lose weight and stuff.

Like Chloe, Anita saw her body as flawed; like Ruth, she cultivated a positive self-perception alongside her personal body critique and the critiques of others. And like Ruth and Chloe, Anita's perception of her body's value did not appear to be the arithmetic result of positive and negative assessments. Her race and build (she was an endomorph in addition to being tall) placed her on the margins of mainstream attractiveness. She experienced her body capital as situational—created in the moment and informed by who was appraising her body, the tone and content of that appraisal, and how she elected to respond. Anita's differed from Chloe and Ruth in that she exhibited stronger resistance to the male gaze and any attendant negative value judgment. She recounted an instance when her father tried to dictate her beverage choice—apparently due to his belief that Anita was not monitoring her calories closely enough:

OK, there was like this one time when like, um, like my dad yell—like me and my dad got in a fight because . . . it was over something stupid too. Like, my dad . . . like, my mom, I think she was . . . saying like that there was—I was asking her what there was to drink 'cause we were eating dinner and like I was ask—asking like for Crystal Light or something and then my mom she's like, "Oh there's juice and there's soda and stuff." And I was like, "Ooo, there's soda!" But . . . I wasn't gonna drink it. And my dad was like, "No, Anita, you can't have soda." And . . . and, um, and he was like, "You have to have water," and I was like, "Well maybe I don't want water." I wasn't, like being—I was just like trying to be funny about it, and then like he yelled at me, "Well, either you have water or you don't have anything at all!" So like, I got pissed at him after he said that, so . . . then . . . when we ate dinner like I didn't wanna eat in the room with them. I ate in the kitchen. They were eating in the dining room and my daddy was like, "Anita, you better eat out here," and I was like, "No, I don't wanna eat out there [chuckles]." So like that was the big thing. And then like, sometimes my dad will like comment on, like one—what I eat and stuff, and um, that's like hurtful.

Ruth joined the track team as a public performance of her attempt to blunt what she perceived as social disapproval of her "fat" body: "So that's why I kind of started doing track. Like, I want people to see that I'm *tryin'.*" Chloe reluctantly resigned herself to delayed desirability: "When they want to, uh . . . like settle down and get married, they look for the smaller girls, I guess." In the above encounter with her father, Anita challenged the province of the male gaze to judge her by literally removing herself from it. This act coexists with her description of her body as "weird" and "hav(ing) meat." It sits alongside Anita's admission that her father's comments about her weight and eating habits were painful. It is therefore inaccurate to conclude that Anita completely embraced the notion of non-size-related beauty, even though she rejected the thin ideal: "I don't wanna be like super skinny, because I think would just look awkward if I was thin, 'cause I'm tall. . . . I have a larger frame also, so like I'm supposed—I'm not supposed to be a size 2, really, like that's what my doctor says." Anita offers yet another example of contingent symbolic body capital. Her practices of self-censure and self-policing responded to the ways her body did not conform to racial, family, or mainstream ideals. She insisted on a certain level of regard for her efforts to present herself well and practice her version of reasonable bodily discipline. She expected others to affirm her efforts and recognize the control limits imposed by her body type.

VALUE AT THE MARGINS INFORMS VALUE AT THE CENTER

These findings lend credence to my assertion that current understandings of African American female body image are informed by a misperception of ethos, and that symbolic body capital within this group is insufficiently explored. The aggregate interview responses and individual narratives are more consistent with an ethos of acceptable personhood than with a broad assertion of indifference to size. Ruth, Chloe, and Anita acknowledged the value assigned to shapely female bodies among African Americans. However, embrace of this familiar norm did not preclude Ruth and Anita's critical self-appraisal of their "fatness" or guard against the emotional pain of others' criticism. The belief that her slender form reduced her dating prospects did not preclude Chloe taking some pleasure in her appearance and abilities. These girls' acknowledgment of particular body norms coexists with a desire to be seen as beautiful as they are by others and with a vulnerability to others' critical looks and comments. The result is a symbolic body capital that is contextually negotiated rather than fixed, patterned by group identity but not predetermined for any individual.

Observing these girls' creative negotiations in the world they have inherited and are reshaping through their engagement with it, we are reminded that our assessments and categorizations of bodies cannot be understood as universal, or even local, truths. "Norm" and "other" are mutually constructing but are not necessarily each other's converse. Identifying something as "not the norm" doesn't explain its nonnormativity or justify its exclusion. Understanding symbolic body capital in US contexts requires not only the recognition that it generally operates differently for white and black women but also that identifying prominent markers of that difference is not the same as understanding the ways the differences are experienced. The current convention of acknowledging and bracketing African American female embodiment as simply "different" neglects that understanding.

The data presented suggest the contingent nature of symbolic body capital among African American females—the symbolic body capital of cultural nondominants in general—merits further exploration. Nondominants' bodies comprise the margins of the body market locally, nationally, and globally. This positioning is neither natural nor accidental: it is the result of historical and currently unfolding processes of meaning and power. As such, bodies on the margin enact divergent, but not completely separate, narratives from those the market favors. This realization brings us back to Du Bois's question and offers yet another modification of it. This further modification links the exploration of nondominant embodied experience to the larger cultural enterprise. "How does it feel to be an exception?" finally becomes "How is value at the margins experienced, and what can that experience tell us about value at the center?"

My findings offer a framework for the explorations that can answer this question. The participants' narratives handily illustrate the emergent nature of symbolic body capital within groups and among individuals (see Becker, this volume) and draw attention to the multiple contexts informing that value. My data and analyses exemplify how the practice of using "the norm" as the basis for defining "the other" tends to obscure complexity and variability. They further suggest that occupying multiple nonreferent categories within a plural society (e.g., not male, not white) further marginalizes nondominant bodies if notions of value are presumed based on "master status" rather than viewed intersectionally. Race-centered value assignment constructs African American female bodies as outside the body marketplace and obscures the range of their embodied experiences. This exclusion and opacity shows itself in that what is likely an acceptable personhood ethos is mischaracterized as a general lack of weight concern. It is discernible in the misreading of a size-inclusive, shape-focused female body aesthetic as a completely size-independent positive body image. It is revealed in the propagation of a racial morphology that strongly links color and size and treats within-race size diversity as anomalous. My research suggests these accepted tenets of African American body culture are misperceptions masquerading as social facts. Exploring the dynamics of body capital among those assigned to the body market margins reveals these misperceptions and invites us to question the pervasive notion of body capital's homogeneity among those closer to the market center.

NOTES

1. Smith et al. (1999) measured three components of body image in their study: Feel-Ideal Discrepancy (a measure of body size dissatisfaction), Appearance Evaluation (a measure of overall weight dissatisfaction), and Appearance Orientation (an indicator of the importance of appearance to the individual and of his/her investment in physical appearance).

2. Grogan (2007) defines body dissatisfaction generally as a person's negative thoughts and feelings about his or her body. Body size dissatisfaction is a person's negative thoughts and feelings about his or her weight.

3. There was one participant for whom African American was not her primary racial identity. However, because she considered African American to be part of her racial identity and she desired to be part of the study, she was enrolled.

CHAPTER SIX

Fat Is a Linguistic Issue

Discursive Negotiation of Power, Identity, and the Gendered Body among Youth

NICOLE L. TAYLOR

Language and materiality are not opposed, for language both
is and refers to that which is material, and what is material
never fully escapes from the process by which it is signified.
—JUDITH BUTLER, *Bodies that Matter*

In *Bodies that Matter*, Butler explores the relationship between language and the body, arguing that the material body is inseparable from discursively constructed norms and power relations. Her analysis provides a compelling rationale for examining not only how discourse influences perceptions about gendered body norms but also the "power relations that contour bodies" (1993, 17). Butler's discussion of the relationships between discourse, power, and the body is wholly theoretical, drawing on poststructuralist, psychoanalytic, and feminist theories (e.g., Foucault, Freud, Irigiray, Kristeva, Lacan). Her theoretically based argument about the connection between language and materiality begs the question: "How do discourse, gender, power, and the body intersect in the material world?"

The body's role in identity formation is particularly salient in the United States, where the perceived ability to control one's body size and shape has an impact on social status, power relations, and even moral identity (Bordo 1993, 1999; Connell 1995; Sobal 1995; Huff 2001; Taylor 2011a). In particular, during the last fifteen years obesity has dominated popular media as one of the most pressing issues of the new millennium. News media focus on obesity as a social, economic, public health, and national security problem—it is commonly referred to as a "crisis" and an "epidemic" and has been framed as a triple threat to our nation by researchers and policy makers who predict that it will take a toll on our economy, health-care system, and military (Boero 2007; Finkelstein et al. 2012; Pace 2006; Charles 2012). The frantic tenor of obesity crisis rhetoric suggests that the problem is urgent but out of our control as a society. And yet the message is clear: we must address this issue before it cripples our nation.

Debate over what causes obesity remains a focal point of public obesity discourses in popular, scientific, legal, and political arenas (Barry et al. 2009; Brownell et al. 2010; Kwan 2009; Leichter 2003; Schwartz and Brownell 2007). A central question underlying the obesity debate is "Who is responsible?" and, by extension, "Who should be held accountable for changing behaviors?" In US popular media, obesity is alternately framed as a public health crisis, an issue of individual and moral responsibility, and a social justice issue (Boero 2012; Brewis 2011; Kwan 2009; Kwan and Graves 2013; Saguy 2013; Saguy, Gruys, and Gong 2010; Saguy and Gruys 2010). Discourses that frame obesity as an issue of personal responsibility and a public health crisis remain predominant, obscuring the everyday realities of discrimination, social inequality, and the pressure to conform faced by those who are labeled overweight and obese (Boero 2012; Kwan and Graves 2013; Puhl and Heuer 2009; Saguy 2013).

Widespread public discourses about the current "obesity crisis" have politicized fatness and highlighted the body's central role in the social negotiation of power relations and identity. Public obesity discourses emphasizing individual responsibility (Lawrence 2004; Kwan 2009), coupled with mass media messages promoting body size as a personal choice (Bordo 1993), have served to reinforce negative stereotypes and social stigma associated with fat bodies. Bordo (1993) argues that mass media messages reinforce the belief about body size as a personal choice through advertisements for dieting products, body-shaping lingerie, exercise equipment, and plastic surgery, leading American consumers to perceive the body's capacity for physical transformation as limitless. In the United States, "body projects" (Brumberg 1997) are central to identity construction, and public discourses about body fat and personal responsibility communicated via mass media are negotiated locally by individuals through everyday discourse and social interaction (Taylor 2011b).

The social meaning of body weight and shape in the United States has shifted throughout history (Bordo 1993; Brumberg 1997; Huff 2001; Sobal 1995; Stearns 2002). Bordo (1993) notes that during the mid-nineteenth century, corpulence symbolized economic prosperity for the bourgeoisie, whereas by the end of the century, "Social power had come to be less dependent on the sheer accumulation of material wealth and more connected to the ability to control and manage the labor resources of others" (192). At the same time, corpulence began to be associated with poor moral character and a lack of willpower.

At the beginning of the twentieth century, health and body-image norms became institutionalized through the medical practice of measuring, weighing, and documenting individuals' body size and weight. By the mid-1900s, insurance companies were using biomedical standards of height and weight to assess morbidity risk in individuals (Huff 2001; Ritenbaugh 1982; Schwartz 1986). This practice further institutionalized a normative standard for body weight as well as the ranking of individuals according to their adherence to this standard. Scholars such as Brewis (2011) offer a more detailed history and critical discussion of how obesity came to be defined and medicalized through measurement of body mass index (BMI) as well as the development of BMI cutoff scores.

Women have long been judged at the site of the body. Fashion and media of the 1920s promoted a slender image of the female body, and a postwar shift in attitude from conservative to carefree prompted women to replace the outward constraint of the corset with the internal constraint of dieting. Movies and fashion magazines began encouraging girls to constantly "try on new identities" through clothing, makeup, and hairstyles. As fashionable clothing for women continued to become more revealing, baring a woman's midriff and thighs, women's focus on body image continued and intensified (Brumberg 1997).

In the 1980s, as diet and fitness industries expanded along with mass media advertisements to sell slimming products, the locus for control and management began to focus more singularly at the site of the body, with consumers responsible for managing their own body weight. As a result, overweight bodies increasingly came to represent laziness, weakness, and a lack of impulse control, whereas thin, toned bodies indexed discipline and willpower (Bordo 1993, 1999; Crawford 1984; Connell 1995; Huff 2001). The emphasis on managing one's body fat that gained momentum during the latter half of the twentieth century increased pressures for boys and men to achieve lean, toned, muscular bodies (e.g., Gill, Henwood, and McLean 2005; Grogan and Richards 2002; Kehler 2010; Ryan, Morrison, and Ó Beaglaoich 2010; Taylor 2011a).

Although dominant body-image ideologies in the United States favor a lean physique and stigmatize excess body fat for both genders (Eisenberg, Neumark-Sztainer, and Story 2003; Griffiths and Page 2008; Neumark-Sztainer, Story, and Faibisch 1998; Puhl and Heuer 2009; Strauss and Pollack 2003), not everyone agrees with or strives to achieve the mainstream beauty ideal. Social science research suggests that body-image ideologies among African American and Latina women may be more flexible than those of white women. Anthropologist Nichter and her colleagues reported that African American teenage girls were more satisfied with their bodies than white girls and defined beauty in terms of attitude, the way one moves, and one's ability to create a personal style that "works" and is unique (Nichter 2000; Parker et al. 1995). A study based on analysis of focus group data similarly reported that African American and Latina women tended to challenge dominant ideals of slenderness, instead embracing an ethic of self-acceptance and nurturance (Rubin, Fitts, and Becker 2003). McClure (2013; McClure, this volume) found a range of body-image satisfaction among African American girls, reporting that their experience with fitness and physicality shaped the way they felt about and presented their bodies.

Beyond the United States, body-image ideals vary cross-culturally depending on the symbolic value placed on body size (Brewis 2011; Gremillion 2005). For example, anthropologist Anderson-Fye found that in Belize women thought body size was God-given and therefore unchangeable. They emphasized body shape and adornment over size, believing that an hourglass Coca-Cola figure was most attractive. Regardless of one's shape, they explained, personal style was key in determining attractiveness (Anderson-Fye 2004). Anthropologists also have reported that larger body sizes, which are considered aesthetically pleasing as well as symbolic of individual health and a thriving community, traditionally have been valued in Jamaica (Sobo 1994) and Fiji (Becker 1995), for example.

Most recently, research suggests a global shift in body-image ideals toward a preference for slenderness. This transition is accompanied by the spread of fat stigma among some non-Western cultures that have traditionally valued larger body sizes. For example, Trainer (2013a) found that modern college women in the United Arab Emirates had embraced Western body-image ideals and reported higher rates of body dissatisfaction than women in their mothers' and grandmothers' generations. Because the processes of this cultural shift are complex, nuanced, and highly dependent upon local contexts, researchers do not yet understand the underlying causal factors (see Hruschka, this volume). However, studies suggest rapid social and economic change, industrialization, and increasing exposure to US media are likely influences (Anderson-Fye 2011, this volume; Brewis 2011; Becker 2004; Becker, this volume).

This chapter explores how adolescents at one US high school co-constructed gendered identities and positioned each other socially through everyday conversation about body image. Body size and presentation played an important role in determining social status among youth in this study. To a certain extent, body size could be manipulated and veiled through clothing and language, creating material and discursive pathways for shifting embodied identities and, consequently, social status. Teenagers positioned themselves as thinner than their peers through clothing, teasing, gossip, and verbal dueling. Regardless of body size, youth discursively shaped perceptions about their own and others' bodies, thereby situating each other in a network of hierarchical relations. In this way, language not only signified materiality but also shaped it, if only momentarily during localized discourse interactions. This chapter explores the tension between efforts to shape body-size perceptions through language and clothing and the undeniable biological reality of body fat.

I draw on the definition of identity that Bucholtz and Hall (2005) articulate: "The social positioning of self and other." This view captures the dynamic nature of identity construction as context sensitive and emergent through discourse interaction as well as relational to co-constructed identities of others, perceived identity categories, and ideological stances. In other words, people negotiate or "try on" identities in specific social contexts and in relation to their perceptions of ideas and individuals with whom they are interacting. Identities that people adopt are changeable in the sense that we experiment with various ways of being but also are enduring in that there are aspects of our identities that may feel essential to the person we perceive ourselves to be in an ongoing way.

I also examine the ways in which youth at this US high school positioned themselves and others through the lens of "disciplinary power" (Foucault 1995 [1975]), a process involving the differentiation of individuals, hierarchical observation, and normalizing judgment. Foucault conceives of disciplinary power as a network of relations among individuals: "Discipline is an art of rank, a technique for the transformation of arrangements. It individualizes bodies by a location that does not give them a fixed position, but distributes them and circulates them in a network of relations" (1995 [1975], 146). This network of relations is both asymmetrical and unstable as individuals negotiate their own and others' positions. Discipline occurs specifically at the site of the body as individuals internalize social norms, self-regulate their behavior and appearance, monitor the behavior and appearance of others, and constantly compare themselves and others against co-constructed norms. Through these internalized, dual processes of hierarchical observation and normalizing judgment, individuals become both the object and enforcer.

Identity co-construction and disciplinary power are primarily achieved through discourse interaction (Bucholtz and Hall 2005; Foucault 1990 [1976]). To provide a concrete example of these processes, the teenagers I worked with negotiated and internalized perceptions about their own and others' bodies by engaging in everyday conversation about body image, gossiping about their classmates' appearance, and teasing each other for transgressing mutually agreed-upon norms related to body size and displays of body fat. Through the constant comparison of themselves and their peers against discursively negotiated body-image norms, adolescents circulated themselves and each other in a network of hierarchical social relations based largely on how they "stacked up" against their peers in terms of physical appearance, which in turn was closely tied to popularity.

METHODS AND SAMPLE

I collected the data analyzed in this article as part of a larger study examining the ways in which sociocultural factors related to weight, including the food environment, food consumption behaviors, participation in physical education classes and physical activity, weight-related stigma, and body-image ideology, intersect in the daily lives of adolescents in a school context (Taylor 2016). Research for this ethnographic study was conducted during the course of one school year at a suburban, primarily middle-class high school I call Desert Vista, located in the southwestern United States. Data collection methods included two individual interviews with each of fifty participants, six focus group interviews, and participant observations throughout the school year in areas where students ate lunch, the girls' locker room, physical education classes, health and life-skills classes, and hallways during passing periods.

The first individual interviews, conducted during the fall semester, lasted about an hour and focused on body-image and weight-based teasing practices. The second individual interviews, which occurred during the spring semester, lasted approximately ninety minutes and focused on diet and exercise. Focus group interviews were less structured than the individual interviews to allow participants to talk more openly about particular topics, such as junk food and advertising, body image and the media, and teasing on campus. Focus groups were comprised of study participants and their close friends—three were all girls, two were all boys, and one included girls and boys. Interview transcripts, interview notes, and field notes were entered into Atlas.ti Qualitative Analysis

Software and coded for emergent themes. Names of participants included in this chapter are pseudonyms to protect confidentiality.

Participants were recruited from the freshman class via physical education classes. I chose freshmen because they had recently made the transition from middle school to high school, where they would have to renegotiate their positions within a broader social context. This renegotiation of social positioning, especially in relation to gendered body-image norms, was a process I wanted to better understand. Following presentations about the study to all freshman physical education classes, I handed out consent and assent forms to students who expressed interest in participating. All students who returned signed consent and assent forms were selected for participation in interviews. I recruited thirty girls and twenty boys, and of the fifty total participants, half identified as white and half identified as Latino or Hispanic, which was somewhat representative of the total high school population at 65 percent white and 30 percent Hispanic.

My research plan focused on examining gender and ethnic differences as key variables in adolescent discourses about body image, food, exercise, and weight-based teasing practices. I had carefully chosen a high school that would allow me to recruit a mix of Latino and white students. What I failed to anticipate was the dissonance in how youth identified ethnically outside the high school setting in their homes and communities and their lived ethnic identities as enacted day to day within the social context of the high school. Soon after I began fieldwork I was surprised to learn that, for teenagers at Desert Vista, the most salient social categories appeared to be gender and social-group affiliation (e.g., jocks, Goths), not ethnicity.

In fact, over the course of the school year, I became increasingly skeptical of the social meaning of ethnicity among adolescents. During interviews, I learned that some participants who initially self-identified as white on the screening form and in the high school social context identified as Latino or Hispanic outside the school context. For example, one girl who had indicated she was white on the screener later told me during an interview that if she could change one thing about the way she looks, she would make her skin lighter because she does not like looking Hispanic. I felt confused as I furtively glanced at her screener and saw that she had indeed identified as white. When I asked the girl why she thought she looked Hispanic, she blushed, looked down at the table, and sheepishly told me she was Hispanic.

Similarly, I learned through an interview with a boy who had self-identified as white on the screener that he really considered himself Latino. His friends on campus were white and so he identified as white at school, presumably to fit in. The boy's grandparents on his mother's side emigrated from Mexico. His mother was Mexican and his father white. At home, his family celebrated quinceañeras, ate traditional Mexican food cooked by his mother, and attended a Catholic church with mostly Latino parishioners. These types of interactions made me question the lived meaning of categories such as "Latino," "Hispanic," and "white." It became increasingly clear to me that students at the high school defined ethnicity through social practice and that it varied depending on context. The lines between socially enacted ethnic identities across family, community, and school contexts were blurred sufficiently that the concept of ethnicity among these adolescents raised more questions than my study on body image and obesity could sufficiently address or incorporate.

Consequently, I realized that if I were to analyze my data according to ethnicity I would have to impose my own categorization onto informants because their perceptions about what it meant to be Hispanic, Latino, or white were neither consistent nor apparent. As an anthropologist committed to foregrounding the voices of the individuals with whom I work, I considered it unethical to impose ethnic labels on these adolescents, many of whom felt conflicted about this aspect of themselves and enacted different ethnic identities depending on the contexts. I also chose not to examine data according to ethnicity because it did not emerge as a salient category for teenagers during interviews. Instead, gender and social-group affiliation were the most meaningful categories to teenagers at Desert Vista. The focus of this chapter is on gender differences in body-image and body-presentation norms.

"PULLING OFF" GENDERED IDENTITIES

I learned during interviews that discursively negotiated and reinforced rules regulating who was allowed to wear particular clothing styles existed for both girls and boys. Participants talked about these clothing rules in terms of who can and cannot "pull off" the fashionable styles. Being able to pull off a style meant wearing clothes associated with the style without attracting negative attention from peers (e.g., getting teased or gossiped about). For boys, pulling off a particular fashionable clothing style was tied to group affiliation, stance or attitude, and social status, whereas pulling off the tight, revealing clothing style that youth deemed fashionable for girls was tied only to body size.

During individual interviews, I asked boys to describe popular clothing styles for boys and girls to describe popular clothing styles for girls. Girls overwhelmingly indicated that "tight" and "revealing" clothes were currently in style. One girl responded, "Right now for girls our age, probably like clothes that show off our midsection and like a lot of cleavage and shorter things." Other responses included the following: "Just tight clothes, like a tight shirt with some tight jeans" and "Like hip huggers that are low and tight and a shirt that's skintight, like really tight." Some explicitly equated tight clothing with femininity. For example, one girl described tight-fitting clothing as "girly" during an interview and reported that people call her a "tomboy" for wearing loose-fitting clothes instead of "girly clothes." Another girl said, "I used to wear a lot of baggy clothes. I used to kind of dress like a guy. And now, lately, I've just been wearing only tight jeans and stuff."

Most boys reported that the "right" fit for guys' clothes is "loose fitting" or "a little baggy." For boys, the ability to pull off certain styles of clothing was based on social affiliation and stance, not body size. For example, in response to a follow-up question about whether or not body size affects a guy's ability to "pull off" certain clothing styles, boys stated that body size was not a factor, often pointing out that they themselves are "small" or "scrawny" but could successfully wear the clothes they deemed stylish. One boy explained, "You've gotta act all big and tough to wear gangster style clothes because people will pick fights with you." Jesse, a tall, thin boy, confirmed that stance was important for "pulling off" his style of clothing, which he described as "gangster," explaining, "It's about like attitude, the way you walk, the way you talk."

Social affiliation also placed constraints on clothing styles that boys were allowed to wear. One boy explained, "You can't wear like real cool clothes and hang with like the nerdy group." Another boy similarly stated that "small," popular boys can wear preppy style clothing but a boy who is not popular, regardless of his body size, will get made fun of for wearing that clothing style. Only boys talked about the tacit rules of boys' clothing styles; no girls commented on boys' clothing styles during interviews except to express jealousy that boys could more easily conceal their bodies under baggy clothing.

In contrast, both boys and girls talked about girls' clothing in terms of who could "pull off" the tight, revealing clothes that adolescents identified as stylish for girls. This commentary was often unsolicited and in-depth, much more than talk about boys' ability to pull off clothing styles. For example, one girl said during an interview that to be able to wear the tight-fitting clothes that are

currently stylish for girls "you definitely have to have a certain type of body."
She explained:

> [Sigh.] You have to be skinny and you have to look good in tight clothes.
> You can't just have everything, like, hanging out. . . . Like, you can't have
> your stomach hanging out cause that just looks bad [laughs]. And you can't
> have your fat showing. It's just not right.

Another girl named Jill told me during an interview that she does not like to
wear tight clothes because she does not think she looks good in them: "I don't
think I have the body for it, so I don't really dress like that. I just wear the
loose stuff." With this statement, Jill displayed her knowledge of the rules about
which girls can pull off wearing tight clothes and acknowledged her choice to
comply by hiding her body fat underneath loose-fitting clothing.

Boys and girls emphasized the importance of girls wearing their proper
clothing size and often went into great detail to describe the appearance of girls
who wore clothing that was too small or too tight. For example, in the context
of talking about girls' clothing during an all-boy focus group, Ricky said that
some fat girls do not know they are fat because they wear clothes that are "too
tight." The other focus group participants responded with comments such as
"It's nasty!" "Once they have a roll it's bad. It squishes out, pops out," and "It's
like cottage cheese."

Similarly, during an all-girl focus group conversation about gossip, the discussion turned to girls who wear clothing that is too small:

MIA: Like you'll see a girl and say, "What was she thinking when she got up
    this morning? Why would she wear that?" I hate it when big girls wear
    little clothes.
JEN: And then it squeezes here and squeezes here [points to thighs] and
    then there's like this chunk just hanging out here [points to midsection].
MIA: They look better if they wear like their-size clothes.

During a mixed-gender focus group, while talking about shopping and girls'
clothing sizes, one boy said, "The thing I hate most when it comes to girls' fashion is the fact of let's say they're supposed to wear like a size 7 or 8 and then they
fit into like a size 3. . . . And then right here they have like all this fat hanging

out." Other participants, both male and female, responded with the following comments: "Yes ugh, ugh"; "It's so gross"; "They have like big ol' fat rolls." At that point, one of the boys in the group pointed to a girl standing nearby and stated that she is an example of a girl who wears clothing that is too tight. The group proceeded to evaluate the fit of her clothing:

EDDIE: Pink skirt [pointing to a girl standing nearby].
KIRA: She's really nice.
EDDIE: I'm just saying.
KIRA: And she's wearing bigger sizes. It's not like she's like trying to wear—
TYLER: She's wearing big sizes because she is big.
LAURA: She's not showing pudge. It's not hanging out everywhere. . . . She's not fat. She's not—
KIRA: She's a little chunky.

Most adolescents, as in the examples above, expressed their views about feminine body-presentation norms through discourse about transgressions. These focus group excerpts also illustrate the ways in which adolescents negotiated female body-presentation norms and their own identities in relation to those norms through everyday discourse about the bodies of their female peers. Interview and observational data confirm that this type of running commentary about the appearance of girls' bodies occurred frequently at school during lunch periods and other times when students gathered in common areas to socialize.

Boys and girls discursively negotiated ideological stances regarding appropriate body presentation for girls and positioned themselves and others in relation to these co-constructed body-image ideals. Just as girls' clothing choices were talked about more frequently than boys' clothing choices and evaluated by both girls and boys, girls who failed to follow the rules for how clothing should fit were gossiped about and teased more frequently than boys who broke the rules because they were subject to surveillance and critique by both boys and girls (Taylor 2011a).

The socialization of body-image norms occurs on many levels. For example, feminist scholars have illustrated the ways in which the advertising of diet products, exercise equipment, and plastic surgery procedures perpetuates and codifies the thin, toned body as normative for women (Nichter and Nichter

1991; Bordo 1993; Brumberg 1997). Everyday discourse is also a powerful vehicle for socialization. Identities, ideologies, and meanings are negotiated and co-constructed moment to moment through everyday conversation (Jacoby and Ochs 1995). In particular, through participation in gossip, girls "increase their stake in the norms, simultaneously tying together the community and tying themselves to it" (Eckert 1993, 35). By engaging in everyday discourse about the bodies of their female peers, girls contributed to their own subjugation, unwittingly presenting themselves for scrutiny by their peers.

These discursive processes were clearly illustrated in the discussions I heard about how girls should present their bodies in clothing. Focus group participants in each of the previous examples co-constructed body-presentation ideals for girls by discursively negotiating mutually agreed upon definitions of what is not acceptable. Through everyday conversations such as these, adolescents co-constructed and reified rules about gendered body presentation, negotiated identities in relation to those rules, reinforced the high school's system of power relations, and positioned themselves and their peers within the social hierarchy.

CONSTRUCTING A "THINNER THAN" IDENTITY

For girls at Desert Vista, having a thin, toned body was a requirement for successfully donning the tight-fitting, revealing clothes deemed fashionable. However, displaying one's flat stomach and thin thighs by wearing low-rise jeans, halter tops, and miniskirts symbolized more than the ability to access fashionable clothing and adhere to a feminine body-image standard. The presentation of taut flesh represented a powerful form of symbolic capital (Bourdieu 1977 [1972]) within the school's social hierarchy.

Girls who could pull off wearing the tight, revealing clothing had higher stature in the adolescent system of power relations. These girls were not only envied by their female peers but also desired and pursued by the most popular boys. Girls who failed to achieve the ideal were considered deviant, especially when they broke co-constructed female body-presentation rules by inadvertently showing their fat in a failed effort to pull off wearing tight-fitting clothing.

For most girls, wearing tight, revealing clothing without showing body fat proved to be an impossible goal due to maturational age, a preponderance of unhealthy "junk" foods in the school setting (Taylor 2011a), and barriers to exercise, such as transportation issues, household obligations, after-school jobs, homework, concern about body appearance during exercise, and social stigma associated with strong, athletic girls. The normative standard against which girls were measured was, in reality, an unattainable ideal, which meant that virtually every girl on campus was perceived and discursively constructed by her peers as deviant. The impossibility of achieving a fat-free body required girls instead to access this form of symbolic capital discursively. Engaging in a daily running critique of their female peers' bodies enabled girls to position themselves as closer to the ideal than other girls.

In mixed-gender groups, when boys initiated critiques of their female peers' bodies, girls often participated because the critical gaze of their peers was diverted away from their own imperfect bodies during that brief interaction. In additional, participating in critiques of other girls' bodies allowed girls to implicitly co-construct their own body presentation as more appropriate and therefore closer to the ideal than the girl being criticized. In this way, the young women positioned themselves and others in relation to a shared feminine body-presentation ideal as well as in relation to each other.

The boundary between thin and fat and between acceptable and unacceptable female body presentation among these adolescents was both discursively constructed and relative. Regardless of their body sizes, they positioned themselves as thinner than their peers through continuous critical discourse about their female peers' bodies. This discourse was largely manifested in negative assessments of how other girls' bodies looked in clothing. Adolescents distanced themselves from the reality of everyday fatness and diverted attention away from their own bodies by calling attention to their peers' fat (Taylor 2011a).

This type of day-to-day discursive negotiation of what constitutes unacceptable displays of body fat also functioned as a tool of disciplinary power within the high school setting, where adolescents were both the object of constant scrutiny and critique as well as participants in that process. In this way, language shaped bodies because it influenced teenagers' perceptions of what looks good, categorizations of their peers in terms of body size and attractiveness, feelings about the way their own bodies looked, and the ways they related to their classmates based on discursively co-constructed perceptions of their body sizes. Through everyday conversations about girls' unacceptable displays of body fat, adolescents co-constructed a perceived "fat" identity category.

Fatness, especially with regard to the female body, is heavily stigmatized in the United States (Nichter 2000; Puhl and Heuer 2009; Brewis 2011), which renders the "fat" identity category undesirable. Adolescents in the present study had internalized public obesity discourses emphasizing personal responsibility for managing body weight as well as the associated negative attitudes and stereotypes about fat people (Taylor 2011b). These youth engaged in continual monitoring of their female peers' bodies and compared themselves and others against discursively negotiated feminine body-presentation ideals through day-to-day conversations about the degree to which their female peers' bodies were perfectly displayed in clothing. This continual monitoring and comparison served to reinforce and police the discursively constructed boundary distinguishing perfect and imperfect feminine body presentation and distribute girls in a network of hierarchical social relations.

Engaging in discourses that focused on girls' body fat enabled adolescents to construct their own identities in opposition to the perceived "fat" identity category. Girls essentially served as the fat foil against which adolescents, both male and female, contrasted themselves as closer to the discursively constructed ideals. Since it was nearly impossible for girls to wear the tight, revealing clothing they deemed stylish and feminine without displaying some amount of body fat, the boundaries of the "fat" identity category were unclear and constantly had to be renegotiated. These shifting parameters meant that almost all girls were potential targets for their peers' critical gaze and could be cast in the role of fat foil.

Girls faced a classic double bind in which they felt strong social pressure to wear tight, revealing clothing but then were punished for doing so. They were forced to choose one of two body-presentation options, neither of which positioned them favorably within the school's social hierarchy. Girls could either wear loose-fitting clothing that hid their body fat and risk being categorized by their peers as "boyish" or they could wear the tight clothing deemed appropriately feminine and risk being teased for displaying body fat. Since virtually every girl was eligible for the perceived "fat" identity category, girls constantly had to position themselves in contrast to this stigmatized identity category through critical discourse of other girls' displays of body fat.

Engaging in this type of discourse interaction enabled girls to negotiate a higher social position, but only within the context of a particular, localized conversation. Because disciplinary power situates individuals as both object and enforcer (Foucault 1995 [1975]), girls had to reassert their "thinner than" identity by engaging regularly in these types of conversations. Groups of adolescents throughout the high school were similarly critiquing the bodies of their female peers, which meant that at the very moment a girl was negotiating a "thinner than" identity by contrasting herself against a fat foil, she herself could be the fat foil for another girl having a similar conversation only a few feet away. Thus the discursively negotiated "thinner than" identity was unstable and fleeting, requiring vigilance and persistence to maintain.

COOPERATIVE COMPETITION AMONG GIRLS

Considering the central role clothing played in how girls were evaluated against the discursively constructed ideal and the bodies of their female peers, it is not surprising that girls expressed a great deal of anxiety around clothing choices. Many of the girls interviewed said they felt pressure to "look cute constantly" and expressed concern about choosing clothing to wear to school, their clothing size as compared to their friends' clothing sizes, and the difficulty of finding clothes that fit "just right." For girls, being able to fit into certain clothes was directly tied to self-esteem. Allie explained during an interview, "Like when you go to a store and you try on clothes and stuff and if they don't fit that makes you feel less confident with yourself and less satisfied with who you are." Similarly, another girl said,

> Well I don't think I'm fat but like . . . you know when you go and try on clothes and you see like the shirt on the little mannequin and you're like, "God it's the sexiest most awesome thing" and you try it on and you're like, "No" . . . and my friends are like, "Do not wear that."

Many girls expressed similar feelings of stress with regard to trying on and choosing clothing to wear.

In addition to the anxiety girls felt while trying on clothing at stores, girls also felt pressure to fit into each other's clothing. Girls explained during interviews that it was common for girls to share and trade clothing. For a girl who wore larger sizes than her friends, this could be an embarrassing and exclusionary social practice. One girl explained:

> My friends, like they wanna either borrow my clothes or like I let them borrow shirts and stuff. But when they wanna borrow pants I don't let

them because none of my pants fit them cause they're [referring to her pants] too big. And when they wanna let me borrow their pants none of them fit me. It brings me down a lot.

Sharing clothing was a marker of group membership among teenage girls. Not being able to participate in clothes sharing with female friends made girls feel marginalized. The seemingly cooperative practice of clothes sharing was in reality fraught for girls who constantly evaluated their own bodies against those of their friends as well as mutually agreed-upon gendered body-presentation ideals.

Girls told me during interviews that they felt pressure to look as good in clothes as their friends did, because the person thought to look the best in tight, revealing clothing occupied a privileged and much coveted place within the adolescent social hierarchy. Girls said that boys flirted most frequently with the thin girls who "wear little bitty clothes." Mia explained:

Angie is like the girl who . . . all the guys like. So like when I go running with her she wears like little tiny wife-beaters [slang for a men's white, sleeveless undershirt] and like these shorts where like her butt hangs out and I feel very uncomfortable running with her. Like I'd rather run by myself and not be compared to her, you know [laughs].

This example further illustrates girls' awareness of being scrutinized by their peers and the pressure they felt to look as good as the other girls in tight, revealing clothing. Mia had internalized and learned to anticipate the male gaze (Mulvey 1975; Goffman 1976; Bordo 1993). And yet the concept of the male gaze does not fully capture what is happening here. These data clearly illustrate the ways in which girls subjected each other to harsh scrutiny and engaged in self-scrutiny as well.

Cooperative competition among girls extended to discourse about body image as well. Girls competed with each other by scrutinizing and critiquing each other's bodies to position themselves as thinner than their female peers. Yet at the same time, girls supported each other through a discourse genre Nichter refers to as "fat talk" (2000). My research supports Nichter's (2000) findings that fat talk serves multiple social functions among adolescent girls, including building rapport, soliciting peer support, calling attention to per- ceived flaws before others do, and aligning with perceptions of feminine norms.

When asked why girls call themselves fat, a majority of girls and boys responded that they are "fishing for compliments." Jen explained, "I think they just want to hear, 'No you're not. You're skinny. You're pretty.'" Similar to Nichter's (2000) findings on fat talk, adolescents I interviewed said the most common replies to a thin or healthy weight girl saying she is fat are "No you're not" and "Shut up." However, in contrast to Nichter's (2000) research, teenagers in my study said that fat girls do in fact engage in fat talk. Students I interviewed said that when fat girls call themselves fat, a prolonged and uncomfortable silence is the most typical response.

One participant explained that she has an overweight friend who sometimes calls herself fat. When she does this, it essentially shuts down the conversation, resulting in an awkward silence, which then is broken by someone in the group who changes the subject. Similarly, a boy described the fat talk ritual among thin girls during an interview, adding, "Sometimes fat girls say that." When I asked him how people respond when a fat girl calls herself fat, he mimicked looking uncomfortable by exaggeratedly looking everywhere but at my face, punctuating this gesture with a prolonged silence.

Conversation analyst Pomerantz (1984) has written that a speaker's assessment of someone or something known to participants invites a response of either agreement or disagreement. According to Pomerantz, "When no overt disagreement is made, the self-deprecating party tends to treat the self-deprecation as implicitly confirmed by the recipient" (1984, 93). Thus, for fat girls at the high school, engaging in fat talk represented yet another vector of critique rather than a means for getting positive feedback from and bonding with other girls.

Clothing and fat talk simultaneously represented sites of competition, rapport building, and support soliciting from girlfriends. However, just as girls who wore larger clothing sizes than their friends were excluded from clothes sharing, fat girls were excluded from participation in fat talk as well, once again placing them at the margins of their friendship groups. Additionally, fat girls who might be labeled as overweight or obese by the majority of their peers also were excluded from discursively positioning themselves as thinner than their female peers, rendering nonnegotiable their places in the adolescent social hierarchy. This circumstance is where materiality becomes undeniable, for very large girls cannot be "not-fat," even through discourse.

Eckert's (1993) research on adolescent girls' interactions indicates that although girls compete to establish status among their peers, they attempt to frame their competition as cooperation because dominant gender norms identify competition with masculinity and cooperation with femininity. Girls at Desert Vista cooperated through sharing clothing, going clothes shopping together, and engaging in fat talk while they competed to look better than each other in clothing—more specifically, to be perceived as thinner than their peers. Girls who were able to discursively construct themselves as thinner than their female peers, regardless of whether or not they could "pull off" wearing tight clothing without displaying body fat, temporarily negotiated a higher status position for themselves.

VERBAL DUELING AMONG BOYS

Even though masculine body-presentation norms required boys to hide their bodies beneath loose fitting clothing, boys remained concerned with how their bodies looked. Virtually all the boys I interviewed said they wanted to be lean, muscular, and have six-pack abs (clearly defined rectus abdominal musculature). In contrast to girls, who masked their body image-related competition in bonding behaviors, such as clothes sharing, boys openly competed with each other over muscle tone, strength, and athletic performance.

Boys gave several reasons for wanting more muscle tone, including improved athletic performance and self-confidence, aesthetics, and a desire to be attractive to girls. Muscle tone was a marker of strength and power, both of which were important aspects of heteronormative masculinity. My findings are consistent with extant research suggesting that boys are, in fact, concerned with how their bodies look and that the heteronormative male body-image ideal is toned, lean, and muscular (Grogan and Richards 2002; Kehler 2010; Ryan, Morrison, and Ó Beaglaoich 2010).

In contrast to early research on boys' body-image ideals suggesting that boys want to develop such large muscles that their bodies would not realistically be able to support the weight of their musculature (Pope, Phillips, and Olivardia 2000), the boys at Desert Vista said there was a limit to how muscular they wanted to be. Several boys from a variety of social cliques cited Arnold Schwarzenegger as an example of someone who was too muscular, with his bulging muscles and veins "popping out." Both boys and girls referenced individuals featured in bodybuilding magazines as examples of what it looked like to be too muscular.

Boys competed with each other directly and in the presence of their peers.

Although some boys claimed to be competitive about athletic ability and clothing brands rather than body image, my interview and observation data suggest that boys were just as competitive as girls about body image. When I asked Kirk, the quarterback of the school's freshman football team, to describe how he and his friends talked about body image, he replied, "Like, 'My six-pack's better than yours' and stuff. It's like a competition." In response to this same question, another boy replied, "It's like, you know, like, 'I'm bigger than you. I'm tougher than you.' That sort of thing."

Jerry, a short, thin, nervous boy who constantly fidgeted during interviews, described a recent conversation he had had with another boy who had claimed to have lifted fifty pounds at the gym the previous day. Jerry responded to the boy by saying, "Yeah, me, too," which he admitted to me was a lie. One girl I interviewed said she had heard guys say to each other, "I can bench press two hundred pounds" or "I have a six-pack." Eder, Evans, and Parker (1995) argue that verbal dueling is a way for adolescent boys to establish a hierarchy among male peers, and they illustrate how physical strength is linked with dominance among adolescent boys. As the examples above suggest, boys at Desert Vista incorporated assertions of physical strength into verbal dueling to negotiate social rank among male peers.

When asked about body-image goals, boys who participated in sports explicitly linked their goal for increased muscle tone with the desire to improve their athletic performance. For example, Kirk, the freshman quarterback who also played basketball and ran track, told me that he wanted "bigger legs" so he could jump higher and "bigger arms" so he could throw farther. Jerry, the nervous, fidgety boy introduced earlier, aspired to be on the school's basketball team. He told me that he wished he were taller, had "bigger calves" and "bigger biceps" to help him perform better in basketball tryouts. These were typical responses among boys who pursued participation in sports.

Most boys admitted that their body-image goals were appearance related as well, reporting that they wanted more muscle tone to feel better about the way they looked and improve their confidence and self-esteem. One boy told me he wanted to start lifting weights "for big arms and everything." When I asked why he wanted big arms, he laughed and said, "Isn't that self-explanatory? It's attractive. It is to me anyway." Another boy said he wanted "stronger biceps" because "it's just kind of almost like a guy thing. I just want stronger arms. It just makes you feel more confident."

Boys also said that girls were attracted to muscular guys, sometimes citing appealing to girls as their main reason for wanting to increase their muscle size and tone. Ricky said during an interview that if he were more muscular he would "get more girls." He explained, "I'd have more friends, too, cause people would be like, 'Aw if I chill with that guy I'll get more girls [laughs].'" Just as girls wanted to look good in tight-fitting clothing to attract boys, boys at Desert Vista wanted well-defined, lean muscles to attract girls. Girls did in fact articulate a strong attraction to boys with lean muscle tone. With the exception of one girl, who said that muscles "don't look good on guys or girls," all of the girls I interviewed said they were attracted to guys with some muscle tone and six-pack abs.

Displaying muscle tone was an important part of constructing a normative masculine identity because it reflected strength and power. One girl said that guys with muscles are attractive "because a guy is supposed to look like he's capable of doing everything." A boy explained that for guys "the goal is muscle because muscle is strength and strength is power." Boys and girls consistently said during interviews that they associated muscles with boys and that muscles did not "look right" on girls. One boy said that guys are not attracted to muscular girls "because girls are supposed to be housewives and ladylike, and muscles don't go with that [image]."

All the boys, with the exception of one, said they would like to have six-pack abs. When I asked boys why, I heard a variety of responses. Many said they liked the way they looked and they thought girls found it attractive: "It [six-pack abs] turns girls on"; "Uh, it just kind of shows, like, a better body, and girls tend to go for better bodies most of the time." Many boys associated six-pack abs with strength: "Girls like boys with six packs because it shows that they are strong"; "It looks very strong and manly." One explained that girls are attracted to guys with six-pack abs because "it just looks good, and, like, girls like to have strong, strong boyfriends. Like, tough usually." The desire for tough, strong boyfriends was widespread among girls I interviewed.

Six-pack abs were a powerful form of "symbolic capital" (Bourdieu 1977 [1972]) at Desert Vista because they reflected strength and power. However, symbolic capital functions differently for adolescent boys and girls within the "heterosexual marketplace" of a high school campus (Eckert 1993; Eckert and McConnell-Ginet 1995). Whereas boys gained status through the display of their own six-pack abs, girls gained status through their relationships with boys who had six-pack abs. Due to female body-image norms disallowing girls to display muscle (or power), most girls did not want to obtain six-pack abs themselves but instead wanted a boyfriend who had six-pack abs.

As I listened to teenagers discuss in detail boys' six-pack abs during interviews, it became clear to me that the adolescents I talked with knew which guys had six-pack abs. I wondered how this form of symbolic capital had become public knowledge when baggy clothing typically covered the stomach. I asked about this during interviews and adolescents explained that boys who have six-pack abs sometimes announced it and lifted their shirts to display their stomachs to peers of both genders.

Tim explained, "If someone has a six-pack, they gotta tell everybody. A lot of times, like, after school, as soon as they get, like, outside the gates out here to the parking lot, they'll, like, take their shirt off and walk around." In this case, the display of symbolic capital in the heterosexual marketplace was more than just a metaphor. Boys were literally advertising their abs for the visual consumption of their peers.

One girl told me during an interview that guys compare their abs by lifting up their shirts and saying, "My six-pack is better than yours" while girls watch. A boy I interviewed explained how guys with six-packs show them off:

NICOLE: How do people know who has a six-pack?
KENNY: When people have a six-pack, they let everybody know.
NICOLE: How do they let people know?
KENNY: They'll just lift up their shirt, and they'll be like, "Yeahhh" [spoken in creaky voice].
NICOLE: Really?
KENNY: Yeah. Or if, like, he's talking to some girl, and then, like, after a while if he wants to impress her or something he'll just show her his six-pack, and she'll be like, "It's so pretty" [spoken in exaggerated high pitch].

Boys displayed their six-pack abs to each other as a means of competing with male peers for status, and they displayed them to girls to attract and impress them.

Whereas clothing fit was most important for girls, boys were more concerned with style and brand name of clothing as markers of social-group affiliation and indices of "coolness." Wearing loose-fitting clothing reflected normative masculinity, which allowed boys to hide their body fat but still feel manly. Loose-fitting clothing had the added advantage of keeping people guessing about how big and strong a boy might be—whether the bulk beneath a boy's shirt was muscle or fat or whether a guy was as scrawny as he appeared or really had lean muscle tone underneath his baggy clothes.

CONCLUSION

This chapter explored how language and materiality intertwine in the daily lives of youth at one high school. For these teenagers, the reality of their material bodies was alternately obscured, reinforced, and challenged through the discursive construction of imagined bodies. Language was the medium through which youth co-constructed identities vis-à-vis gendered body-presentation norms and circulated themselves and each other in a network of power relations. Body image and, by extension, gendered identities were co-constructed discursively as youth positioned themselves in relation to each other through contrasting themselves against perceived body-presentation transgressions of their peers and aligning themselves with body-presentation ideals. The circulation of discourse about girls' body-presentation transgressions and boys' six-pack abs, real or imagined, functioned as a tool of disciplinary power.

Yet language does not tell the whole story. The physical reality of the body, the materiality that Butler (1993) refers to in the opening quote, cannot be denied. Adolescents at Desert Vista were constantly butting up against the physical reality of their bodies. The ultimate goal for most teenagers, boys and girls, was to eradicate visible body fat. Boys wanted lean muscle tone and six-pack abs, and girls aimed for thin overall physiques with flat stomachs. However, they could not escape the biological reality that every body contains fat. Some adolescents could approach the body-image ideal to varying degrees, but none could achieve the so-called perfect body. This unattainable goal is, in fact, the nature of an ideal—it is something one strives for but never quite achieves.

Not only were students at Desert Vista unable to achieve the ideal, but many of those I interviewed were overweight and a few were obese, which generally reflected national BMI trends for youth. In the context of this material reality, teenagers focused on strategically hiding their fat beneath clothing. The popular style for boys was loose-fitting clothes, which made obscuring fat relatively easy. However, it was nearly impossible for girls to wear the tight, revealing outfits considered stylish and feminine without displaying some amount of body fat.

This meant that almost all girls were potential targets for their peers' critical gaze and could be cast in the role of fat foil.

Even though the majority of Americans are categorized medically as overweight or obese, fat-free body-image ideals remain predominant in the United States. As youth have become larger, they increasingly are unable to display bodies that approach dominant gendered body-image ideals. This trend may further highlight the role of language in constructing gendered bodies. Youth in the present study used language to shape perceptions about their own and others' bodies and thereby situate each other in a network of hierarchical relations. In this way, language not only signified materiality but also shaped it, if only momentarily during localized discourse interactions.

CHAPTER SEVEN

Body Size, Social Standing, and Weight Management

The View from Fiji

ANNE E. BECKER

The conceptual framing of body weight as responsive to personal volition and practice is a half-truth (Friedman 2004) with historic and globally broad success. There is something intransigent about this fiction, which has gained immense traction both in the United States and in many other regions of the world. This particular frame positions body weight as a symbolic reservoir with opportunities for modulation that can be used to contrive a desired personal narrative on the one hand, or, when neglected, to invite disdain on the other. Whereas the cosmetic sleight of hand to *inscribe* or dress the body takes so many forms it is difficult to recount an exhaustive inventory, the punishing and recalcitrant domestication of the body through weight management may have uniquely adverse health and social consequences.

The backdrop for this chapter is the global rise in obesity prevalence, which is undisputed, even if the causal factors remain both opaque and contested (e.g., McGarvey 1991; Popkin 2001; Brownell and Horgen 2004; Friedman 2004; Marcus and Wildes 2009; Flegal et al. 2012). Pacific Island populations have been famous for both exceptionally high obesity rates (Bindon and Baker 1985; Brewis et al. 1998; Duarte et al. 2003; Hodge et al. 1994; Hodge et al. 1995; Metcalf et al. 2000; Coyne 2000; Tomisaka et al. 2002) and storied counterfactual body ideals (Mackenzie 1985; Becker 1995; Ben-Tovim 1996). Evidence also indicates an increase in these already high rates in several of these Pacific populations (Duarte et al. 2003; Hodge et al. 1994; Flegal 1999; Ulijaszek 2001), including in Fiji (Becker, Gilman, and Burwell 2005). The fallout from this epidemic is measured not only in its well-substantiated impact on a broad swath of non-communicable diseases (National Food and Nutrition Centre 2007; Dalton and Crowley 2000) but also by the attendant social misery of stigma (Gortmaker et al. 1993; Hebl and Mannix 2003; Friedman 2004; Puhl, Andreyva, and Brownell 2008; Puhl and Heuer 2009). Socially sanctioned derision and stigmatization of fatness have been recognized and critiqued in the usage of terms such as *fat talk* and *weightism* in the professional literature regarding eating disorders for decades (Steiner-Adair 1978; Nichter 2000), where the deleterious health and social impacts of socially normative disparagement of overweight (Britton et al. 2006) are well cataloged (Sharpe et al. 2013). Likewise, the stigmatization of obesity warrants interrogation for many reasons, not least because it is not always inadvertent (Martin 2010; Puhl, Peterson, and Luedicke 2013).

If body-shape and -size ideals encode core cultural values, weight may well be an overdetermined reservoir for social meanings. It is not difficult to see, moreover, how body-size aesthetics track with collective sensibilities regarding prestige, as well as the veneration of self-cultivation as examined in a vast literature on body and self (e.g., Goffman 1959; Lasch 1979; Bourdieu 1984; Foucault 1988; Giddens 1991; Bordo 1993; Turner 1984). Numerous examples illustrate the historical and cross-cultural variation in the lexicon of body-size and -shape ideals (Mackenzie 1985; Becker 1995; Pope, Phillips, and Olivardia 2000), even if globalizing commerce, travel, and communication platforms now more broadly distribute exposures that overwrite local social norms (Becker 2004; Becker et al. 2011). Indeed, the scientific literature on eating disorders tells the story of a one-two punch exposing young women to an elevated risk of eating pathology when they undergo social transition (for example, due to migration, urbanization, or rapid regional economic development), while also encountering historically Western postmodern social pressures to be thin (Striegel-Moore and Bulik 2007; Becker et al. 2010b; Gerbasi et al. 2014). Setting aside some interesting and unresolved debate in the literature on the relation of acculturation to eating pathology, this particular narrative about exposure and risk assumes a rather narrow corridor of influences connecting the social valuation of thinness to body dissatisfaction, pursuit of thinness, and disparagement of fatness. Likewise, in the obesity literature, personal agency in weight (and self) management has been curiously naturalized in both biomedical and folk models of fatness. This oversubscription to personal agency in weight control, in part, underwrites both the valorization of thinness and the stigmatization of obesity. In contrast, the metastory of body-ideal changes in Fiji provides a context for a deeper examination of the relations among local social values, migrating body-size ideals, and weight stigma.

A SHORT AND RECENT HISTORY OF
BODY-IDEAL CHANGES IN FIJI

In the mid-1990s broadcast television was established in Fiji, a nation located in Oceania. The programming featured content that was mostly produced in the United States, Australia, New Zealand, and the United Kingdom and thus imported and circulated many new ideas. A pilot study exploring the impact of these novel exposures through television provided sentinel findings of a shift in female body-size ideals in Fiji—specifically from the traditionally preferred robust body toward the thinner size represented in many of the locally available television shows. In this ecological study, a snapshot comparison between a cohort of young women in 1995 and a second, matched cohort in 1998 bore evidence of what might be viewed as a surge in disordered eating over this relatively short span of time (Becker 1995; Becker et al. 2002; Becker 2004). Apart from the ominous relevance of this shift to the mental health of young women in Fiji, the migration of body-weight ideals is both an illustration of how body shape and size encode core social values and an exemplar of their marvelous fluidity.[1] A similar transition—from a preference for rotund, more corpulent body shape through the twentieth century in the United States to a comparatively slender figure—has been elegantly documented (Brumberg 1989). Notwithstanding some oddly chosen metrics and proxies for this shifting ideal—*Playboy* centerfold bust, waist, and hip measurements, for one—an aesthetic of thinness became standardized against relatively prominent benchmarks in the visual mass media (Garner et al. 1980; Silverstein et al. 1986), routinized, and entrenched in the latter decades of the twentieth century.

This slow march toward a new slender ideal seemed to converge with data suggesting that transnational migration, urbanization, and assimilation to Western values, images, and ideas were associated with the high valuation of slenderness. This valuation was sometimes associated with dieting and eating pathology in other populations and regions of the world. The globalization of eating disorders, moreover, is consistent with recently published Global Burden of Disease Study data, demonstrating in excess of a 65 percent increase in the estimated health burden attributed to eating disorders between 1990 and 2010 around the world (Murray et al. 2012). Additional data from a large and representative sample of school-going Fijian girls (study methods described in Becker et al. 2009) demonstrated that eating pathology had become even more prevalent by 2007. Of the 523 adolescents in that study, 42 percent reported purging or the use of herbal purgatives in the preceding month. Although latent profile analysis supported the clinical salience—as measured by distress and impairment—associated with these behaviors (Thomas et al. 2011), the patterns proved culturally distinctive and perplexing. Approximately half of the young women who reported purging also reported taking indigenous remedies for *macake*, an indigenous illness characterized by loss of appetite (Becker 1995). Moreover, although some of the young women purged in secret, others collaborated with their mothers or other family members as if their weight were being co-managed. Although the disordered eating had all the earmarks of purging behaviors that adversely affect health, it did not align with familiar presentations of eating pathology described in the fourth edition of the *Diagnostic and Statistical Manual of Mental Disorders* (DSM-IV) (APA 2000). It is therefore informative to contextualize them within Fiji's rapid and dramatic social changes.

DIET, BODY WEIGHT, AND SOCIAL HEALTH IN FIJI

Body-size ideals in several Pacific Islander societies have been described in the literature as notable for their contrast with the late twentieth-century slender and toned body ideals in North America. In some instances, fatness was fetishized for women as a marker of high social status. In late-twentieth-century Fiji, traditional preferences also marked large body size as a salient positive attribute for both males and females. This preference for robust body size was linked fairly explicitly to its representation of social health (Becker 1995; Mavoa and McCabe 2008). For example, a large—and well-fed—body was tangible evidence of a robust social network with the means and inclination to care for its members well.

To give just one illustration of how social values can be encoded in body shape along multiple, independent dimensions, survey data on iTaukei Fijian preferences for body size were collected among a mixed-age, community-based sample of men and women (n = 301) in the late 1980s. The respondents were asked to rate twelve drawings of adult female bodies depicting a range of adiposity along a spectrum from very underweight to obese (labeled A–L and shuffled and presented in random order) along dimensions of attractiveness and perceived quality of care being received. Although attractiveness and quality-of-care ratings demonstrated correspondence in negative valuations of the thinnest shapes (A–C) and in positive valuations of medium shapes (D–G), they diverged for the largest size shapes (I–L) in modal ratings *simultaneously* reflecting that the heaviest shapes were perceived as both the *least* attractive and the *best* cared for among the range of shapes (Becker 1995). In other words, modal ratings for attractiveness followed an inverted U-shaped curve along the spectrum of thinness to fatness, where the least-preferred shapes were at those two extremes. In contrast, modal ratings on the dimension of care received associated the thinnest shapes with least well cared for and the fattest shapes with most well cared for.

These quantitative data were consistent with ethnographic data indicating that body size concretizes care from the family and broader social network. Care itself is a multidimensional construct in Fiji, with the prominent dimension, *viqwaravi*, denoting feeding, serving, and tending to the needs of a guest or family member. Bodies, then, are the responsibility and achievement of the family or social network that feeds them. This principle is also visible in what might be a scathing critique of a family that fails its members by allowing them to go thin or by not responding to signs of macake, including appetite loss. Many other illustrations of the social appropriation of bodies exist in the etiologic attribution of illness to social disharmony (Becker 1995; Becker 1998) and the occasional repurposing of individual bodily space as a vehicle for public messaging (e.g., as seen during a possession by a *yalo ni cala*, a spirit concerned with wrongdoing). Conversely, the possibility of an elopement of bodily secrets (such as in the well-recognized extracorporeal manifestations of an undisclosed pregnancy; Becker 1997) situates the body in social space. This point is worth dwelling on since the body's location in social space subverts an assumption of personal agency, including personal responsibility for body weight in Fiji, which has arguably become naturalized in American culture.

Of course, "American culture" is no more monolithic and static than iTaukei Fijian culture. That said, it is useful to hone in on prominent social values carried in mainstream contemporary American culture as a heuristic in understanding how social values are manifest in body practices and otherwise embodied. Nor are these practices unique to mainstream American culture. Indeed, social pressures to be thin have infiltrated mainstream discourse in areas of Europe, South and Latin America, East Asia, and the Antipodes. The uptake of the pressures to be slim varies, however; for the purpose of highlighting contrasts, we will focus on peculiarities in mainstream contemporary American culture. In the United States, the valorization of thinness appears to be at a pole on one end of a spectrum that is anchored on the other with a derision of fatness. The

brilliant commercial success of the weight-loss industry—in the face of stag-
geringly high recidivism of overweight—may be the clearest proxy measure of
the conviction that personal effort can override formidable barriers to weight
maintenance. Moreover, socially sanctioned aspirations for achievement and
exceptionalism render body-shape ideals fair targets for self-improvement and
upward social mobility.

DIET AND HEALTH IN FIJI

There are several prominent socially salient dimensions of dietary quality in Fiji.
First and foremost, access to and receipt of high-quality and abundant food is a
marker of respected social status. This respect (*varokotaki*) and care (*vikawai-
taki*) are both evident in process indicators (for example, in invitations to dine;
food gifts; attentive hosting, or viqwaravi; or serving notably abundant, diverse,
and high-status foods such as yams, sweet potatoes, taro, roast pork, and turtle)
and in their concretization in robust body size (that can be described as *levulevu vina*) and growth (favorably described as *jubu vina*). In these respects,
dietary quality is, in fact, constituted by social interactions that both recognize and enhance esteem. That is, the appraisal of diet quality is not linked
explicitly to nutritive content but indexes the quality of social interactions and
social status. Traditionally, the components of a high-quality meal related to
balance between two food categories: *na cawa dina* and *na kea ilava*. Literally,
these translate to "real food" and "its accompaniment." These terms refer to
the dietary foundation of starchy root crops (e.g., taro, cassava, sweet potatoes,
and yams) and a relatively smaller amount of fish or meat, often prepared with
added fat, such as coconut cream. As in the socially constructed—and ever
changing—food pyramid so familiar to US consumers, the importance of balance from major food groups is emphasized. However, foods in Fiji are locally
categorized within a different classification scheme. Green and yellow vegetables are often served with an apology, and fruits are regarded as snack foods,
not integral to meals. Although the ideal Fijian diet happens to be calorie dense
and macronutrient rich, its rationale is socially derived rather than aligned with
biomedically informed nutritional guidelines.

SOCIAL VALUES, CARE, AND "OVEREATING"

Social values are conspicuously performed and affirmed during routine meals as well as rather frequent feasts (*magisi*) given that serving and consuming an abundance of food concretizes mutual respect. In addition to the distribution of specific foods, both the geography of the table and timeline of the service recognize and reify the social hierarchy of attendees. Care, or viqwaravi, is performed in hosting a meal, when guests or family members are invited to partake of the best foods at the table and could even be seen to be coached on eating abundantly. The rhetoric of mealtime coaching might even include playful insults, such as "You are eating like a nurse" ("O iko kana vanasi"), referencing a pattern of eating with uncharacteristic self-restraint. Consistent with traditional values, the opportunity to eat beyond physiologic satiety was previously regarded as a fortunate and pleasant social circumstance. However, over the past two decades, some young women have begun to experience and comply with expectations to consume heartily at feasts in a different manner. They remain keenly aware of the social pressures to eat an abundant quantity of food. They also enjoy the special foods typically served at feasts. Nevertheless, some experience shame associated with publicly eating a large amount of food, whereas others worry about excessive weight gain. In this respect, their discomfort stems from emerging dissonance between traditional and contemporary values, the latter manifesting for now in the infiltration of stigma into excessive food consumption.

THE SOCIAL CONSTRUCTION OF OVEREATING

If fat is stigmatized partly as a proxy of unrestrained eating, it is fruitful to interrogate how "overeating" is socially constructed. Embedded in the term in English is the deviation from social norms, connoted by the prefix *over-*. The problem here, of course, is that normative eating is highly variable across not just geography, but also time, season, and social circumstances.

Understanding the dimensional nature of eating (under- or over-) is also integral to deconstructing how deviation from socially normative eating can be classified as binge eating. As research criteria for binge eating disorder (BED) in the DSM-IV (APA 2000) were considered for revision and elevation to diagnostic criteria in the DSM-5, questions arose about the clinical operationalization of binge eating. As published in the DSM-IV, the standing definition rested on two relatively subjective dimensions—eating more than what most people would, given the social circumstances, and loss of control of how much one ate. Clinical researchers, moreover, could discern that many respondents experienced "subjective binge episodes" that did not meet the usual clinical standard for "objective binge episodes" insofar as the consumption that may have felt large to the respondent was not judged to be large by clinicians. This discrepancy possibly stemming from cognitive symptoms associated with the presentation of eating disorders, is also plausibly due to socialization to varying norms for portion size. Nonetheless, it seemed salient that respondents indicated they experienced "loss of control" during these episodes, raising the question of whether it mattered that only a small or moderate amount of food was consumed (e.g., see Vannucci et al. 2013).

As part of the scouring of scientific literature and empirical data that would inform the clinical diagnostic criteria and guidance for the DSM-5, Wolfe and colleagues (2009) conducted a scientific review of representative studies of binge *size* in bulimia nervosa. It is important to note that the operational definition of a binge episode was consistent across the diagnostic categories, bulimia nervosa and binge eating disorder (APA 2000). Yet the range of calories consumed during a binge varied as much as fifty to one hundred times within some studies—for example, from 52 to 5,465 Kcals (Rossiter and Agras 1990) and from 1,000 to 55,000 Kcals (Johnson et al. 1982). These extraordinary ranges reveal a critical finding: neither social norms nor a clinical consensus easily captures the definition of the term *binge*.

Relevant to this discussion is how the loss of control is configured and morally valenced against local norms. For example, positing a loss of control implies preexisting control—that is, autonomy and agency over dietary options and choices. Autonomy and agency are typically assumed for American adults and are in fact intentionally modulated in the service of therapeutic goals in treating binge eating (e.g., in residential treatment settings where meals and postmeal bathroom visits might be supervised and kitchen cabinets may be locked). In a typical Fijian household, responsibility for procuring and offering meals substantially lies with others. Similarly, a lack of privacy or even food insecurity also can constrain an individual's decisions and opportunities to consume a large amount of food. In such contexts, the starting point for "normative" self-control is very different—as are departures from it. Further, nonsharing of food in Fiji is stigmatized, illustrated by the insult *kanakana lo*, a derogative term to describe someone who does not share food (literally, "one who eats secretly"). On the other hand, the Fijian idiom *kana variva* (to eat crazily) does not have a clearly negative moral valence, since presumably the eating is wrapped into a moment of social exchange of care and food.

OVEREATING AND STIGMA

Even in contexts in which control over eating is generally perceived as within the domain of personal choices and flexible options, the social construction of "loss of control" eating acknowledges a range of driving influences, including both external "triggers" and the interior spaces of neuro-circuitry. For example, in *Almost Anorexia*, where Thomas and Schaefer (2013) chart the gray area between socially normative discontent with body, weight, and food and clinically recognized eating disorders, they refer to a societal "voice" — "societal Ed" — that can be experienced as intruding into and residing in one's "head." Substantial empirical data, on the other hand, demonstrate that appetitive drive is regulated by complex, if still poorly understood, satiety hormones and neuro-transmitters. Notwithstanding these formulations of ways in which appetite and dietary consumption are governed by social and biological mechanisms, there is a persistent misattribution of self-agency over diet and weight that legitimates the stigma attached to perceived failures to self-regulate weight (Becker 2013). The dimension of "loss of control" over eating might arguably be seen to be especially pathologized and stigmatized in contexts in which control is both valued in itself and can be seen as integral to achievements that are socially desirable (such as are reflected in educational attainment or physical fitness).

At the same time, tremendous variation exists in perceptions of proxies for overeating — for example, fullness. We understand from the scientific literature linking gastrointestinal symptoms to measurable pathology (such as delayed gastric emptying or slowed intestinal transit) that the alignment between subjective report (i.e., what patients experience as symptoms) and measureable gastrointestinal dysfunction (i.e., what physicians take to be signs) is imperfect and highly variable (Becker and Baker 2010). The gap between what is experienced and what is measurable is likely to be best explained by variable socialization toward normative experience: for example, is it good to feel full? And if so, what is a good amount of fullness? Is it good or is it noisome to feel hungry? What does it mean to feel hungry? Is this an achievement or an alarm?

When the National Comorbidity Survey Replication data on eating disorders were published in 2007, the findings belied clinical understandings of what the prevalence and course of disordered eating looks like in a representative community sample. What can be gleaned from that study is not just that eating disorders frequently come and go without ever formally declaring themselves in clinical settings, but also that the experience and emotional valence of binge behavior appears to be highly gendered. Curiously, Hudson and colleagues (2007) found, that although the lifetime prevalence of BED was significantly higher among women than men, subthreshold binge eating disorder (described as principally differing from BED in the absence of distress associated with the binge eating) was significantly more prevalent in men. This gender discrepancy—between binge eating associated with and without distress—makes a categorical difference in assigning a diagnosis of BED. Nevertheless, it does not change other phenomenologic similarities in binge eating between women and men in the United States, even if distress about overeating or losing control over eating may be moderated by gender. One plausible interpretation of this finding includes that men are not as distressed as women are by their binge eating because of differences in perceived deviation from social norms.

Returning to the story in Fiji, narrative and ethnographic data illuminate the dissonance potentially experienced by young women as they navigate the expectation that they conform to social etiquette by eating abundantly at feasts and a growing social critique and public commentary about overeating. Eating well into satiety was previously recognized as mutual achievement at a meal—evidenced in a typical exchange, "Eat a lot" (*kana valevu*) or "Eat again" (*kana tale*) and the standard closing response, "I am really sated" (*qi bori hara ga*)—and indeed, a social obligation (Becker 1994; Becker 1995). More recently, however, the moral salience of overeating appears to be in flux. This reversal is stunningly evident in remarks published in the *Fiji Times* newspaper in 2014 (Sauvakacolo 2014):

> CONCERNS over the excessive consumption of kava, tobacco and *food* [emphasis added] have led to strict monitoring of its use during funeral proceedings of former Methodist Church of Fiji president Reverend Tuiki-lakila Waqairatu.

Moreover, the Fiji Methodist Church's communications secretary, Reverend James Bhagwan, was quoted as saying,

> The biblical understanding from the late president was that the body was the temple of God and that referred to kava, tobacco, *over-eating* which are all forms of substance abuse. (Sauvakacolo 2014; emphasis added)

SOCIAL CHANGE, SOCIAL MOBILITY, AND WEIGHT IN FIJI

Rapid economic development over the past few decades in Fiji has transformed the country's infrastructure of economic and social opportunities. Although it is impossible to catalog these changes and their cascade of impacts exhaustively, notable changes exist that are relevant to the migration of body-weight ideals and their relevance to social mobility. If we were to take Fijian convention and ideology as bedrock, there would be little recognized formal opportunity for upward social mobility in Fiji. In theory, educational achievements have been an established pathway toward highly respected professions in the health, education, and civil service sectors, social standing and privilege are also firmly linked to chiefly lineage. Traditional authority likewise has been vested with chiefs, and chiefly governance continues in formally recognized ways. Conventionally, social status in Fiji is closely aligned with lineage, birth order, and gender (Ravuvu 1983). Chiefly status, for example, is a legacy of both parents, although the patriline figures more prominently. Membership in a chiefly *mataqali* (clan) likewise confers high status. Opportunities to highlight chiefly lineage or social ties (through naming with the honorific prefixes of *Ratu*, *Adi*, or *Bulou*, for example) exist, but this important dimension of the social hierarchy still is rather fixed at birth. As a result, mapping a personal trajectory toward upward social mobility is not particularly valued traditionally and can even be fraught with social danger (Becker 1995).

In contrast, novel opportunities to find wage-earning occupations and migrate to towns and urban areas appear to offer new pathways for young people to define and achieve alternative goals. Earlier data showed that young women were attuned to narratives of successful navigation of opportunities and jobs depicted in television dramas imported from the United States, Australia, New Zealand, and the United Kingdom. They explicitly noted their interest in characters who had found employment, expressed admiration for their lifestyle, and articulated a desire to emulate it (Becker 2004). This shift in ambition is illustrated vividly in contrasts between study participants' aspirations and parental achievements occupationally in table 7.1. That is, the vast majority of 2007 respondents—young iTaukei women between the ages of fifteen and twenty attending secondary schools across a swath of coastal and rural, inland locations—endorsed a desire to enter a professional occupation whereas fewer than 2 percent planned to work within the more traditional agrarian and domestic household roles the majority of their parents held. Approximately half of these

Table 7.1. Participant-reported parental and aspirational occupations (n = 523).

	Parental occupation (%)	Respondents' aspirational occupation (%)
Agrarian and domestic labor	62.4	1.34
Retail, service, other unskilled labor	21.3	18.40
Professional occupation	16.2	79.50

students attended secondary schools in rural areas and half attended schools within or near a town with a population of approximately ten thousand. A similarly revealing juxtaposition is that, whereas a modest majority reported household ownership of a television in the household, nearly the same percentage reported residence in a household without at least one of the following: running water, electricity, refrigeration, or a gas stove.

Notably, measures of perceived feasibility of upward social mobility, as well as personal ambition for it, were significantly and moderately correlated with Western/global cultural values ($r = .263$ and $r = .317$ respectively; $p < .001$ for both) but not with iTaukei Fijian values ($r = .058$ and $r = .054$; $p = $ NS; Becker et al. 2010a). Taken together, ethnographic, narrative, and epidemiologic data in Fiji suggest a phenomenologic shift in the texture and horizon of social aspiration of young iTaukei Fijian women amid this rapid economic transition. The pathway for adolescent girls into adulthood had been girded by social caste and gender and governed by expectations and social sanctions inhering to rigid social hierarchies. By 2007, however, expanded access to educational and wage-earning opportunities had overwritten previous economic constraints to upward social mobility.

TELEVISION, SOCIAL CHANGE, AND
UPWARD MOBILITY IN FIJI

Given these changes, it is not difficult to understand why young women found television drama narratives so compelling when Western-produced programs first came to Fiji. The impact of television's debut there may have been overdetermined in that it could not have arrived without the infrastructure that carried many other vehicles of social and economic development. Imported televised programming in Fijian homes unfolded in a context of global capital investments in tourism that required such infrastructural upgrades, for example, and provided additional exposures to Western products, lifestyles, and ideas. In many ways, television content provided a quintessential view into a globalizing consumer culture that also was making cameo appearances via the print media, the encroaching tourism industry, and various relatives who crossed the Coral Sea south to New Zealand or Australia, and then back, in order to seek jobs. Television ignited the imaginations of young women who were keenly interested in how the adolescents in *Beverly Hills 90210*, to name one example, landed employment. Accustomed to public scrutiny and discussion of body size and weight, they keyed in on the slenderness of the actresses on television. They also remarked on the near ubiquity of thinness and started aspirational patter regarding how they could emulate TV characters who navigated employment and affluence so well. Their expressed admiration was not strictly around aesthetics—although it might be argued that social prestige infuses aesthetics in ways that make the two difficult to distinguish. They also admired the character Xena (from *Xena: Warrior Princess*), whom they viewed as strong and powerful. For instance, one of the respondents commented that she saw Xena as validating that women could be powerful too. The young women looked to television characters and narratives as guideposts. They specifically commented that they studied the characters—even the characters on the *X-Files*—to discover how to steer their lives toward similar appealing goals (Becker et al. 2002; Becker 2004).

Television narratives were only one of several novel vistas that suffused the aspirations of Fijian girls with ideas that departed from the expectations of their parents' and grandparents' generations. Among these was the possibility of authoring a new and different life script. Whereas the majority of young women in rural Fiji had parents who worked in traditional domestic and agrarian roles, the overwhelming majority of these young women aspired to a more prestigious or remunerative occupation. This ambition may have stemmed from their parents' encouraging them to find employment that could generate or subsidize family income. It could also have been driven by their own generation's ideas about what navigation would be necessary to enjoy a good life. Regardless of the reasons, the young women evidenced broad ambitions regarding educational and occupational goals. During this era, and to the consternation of the adult generation, adolescent girls seized greater autonomy—perhaps most visibly manifest in departures from prescriptive conformity to traditional social norms for dress, hairstyle, and weight management (Becker 1995).

The plasticity of body-size and body-shape ideals, as well as their polyvalent meanings and moral attributions, are relevant to understanding how body size is perceived and even used as a means of competitive social positioning (see also Anderson-Fye 2004; Anderson-Fye et al., this volume). Although control over fatness tends to be naturalized in mainstream American culture (despite a strong counternarrative in the scientific discourse on the biological grounding of defense of body weight in regulation by satiety hormones, the microbiome, etc.), this is not the prevailing attitude in Fiji. Authority and responsibility for body weight and size are located within the extended family and, sometimes, the community. As with social status, which is—at least conventionally—fixed at birth, body weight is not a dimension of self that is amenable to social mobility. As the spectrum of social opportunities in Fiji has enlarged to encompass wage-earning jobs, accessible via avenues other than birthright, young women have begun to perceive the possibility of new life trajectories. They see that education, effort, and competent navigation of a Westernizing landscape might lead to new opportunities for social and economic success—a concept that has not been lost on their parents, either.

Although deeply situated in a personal history, ambition is also a collective enterprise in Fiji and families likewise recognize the economic stakes attached to emerging opportunities within the modernizing social landscape. On the one hand, young women wish to pursue appealing economic opportunities. On the other, mastery of necessary competencies, and their successful deployment, may place young women in conflict with prevailing social and moral norms that their primary allegiance be to family and community. Consistent with the conventional Fijian location of feeding and body-weight management within the family matrix, evidence shows that young women in Fiji seek to align their weight-management goals with these plural social values and norms. Examples of the calibration (or recalibration) of weight goals and co-management of weight with family support illustrate how body weight is a socially—not personally—authored venture. Interestingly, excerpts from interviews with young women participating in the aforementioned study (Becker et al. 2009) reveal their perception that fatness is stigmatized and a potential barrier to social and economic opportunities. For example, a respondent who used herbal purgatives answered interview questions as follows:[2]

I: And do you feel different if you're thinner or slimmer?

s: Yes.

I: And how, what would you feel like?

s: I'd not be my own self and I would be like doing other stuff that I wasn't doing before. Like hanging around with cool kids.

I: . . . Do you think that it would influence what kind of job you would get?

s: Yes.

I: What do you want to do?

s: I want to become an air hostess. (I-12)

Another study participant's responses revealed her connecting weight to social standing among friends:

I: And what does your family think about it?

s: They think that I should lose weight too.

I: Why do they think that you should lose weight?

s: Because I'm, like, fat.

I: But what do they think would be different if you lost weight?

s: I would be, I mean, I would get lots of friends. And they won't be treating me like this.

I: What about other things outside of friends, what about jobs? Do you think that size and shape influences that?

s: Yeah, sometimes.

I: When?

s: Like, air hostess.

I: Air hostess? Do you want to be an air hostess?

s: Of course, yes. They only want slim girls.

I: How do you know that?

s: One of my friends told me.

I: So why do they want slim girls?

s: I don't know. Maybe to walk easily into the plane. (I-28)

The quest for upward social mobility for this young women is complicated by its juxtaposition with expectations of selfless service to one's community. With development of the tourism industry, largely concentrated in coastal and urban areas, entry into wage-earning jobs in the tourism sector may require rural inland villagers to relocate. Enrollment in choice schools or pursuit of tertiary education may necessitate a move into urban areas. For others, job opportunities draw them to relative windfall opportunities overseas in high-income countries, including Australia, Canada, New Zealand, and the United States. The accrual of wealth can generate tensions upon reentry, however. Fijian traditions virtually mandate some sharing of traditional material wealth and food, but these cultural expectations have more vague and tenuous traction for cash or goods acquired in the commercial sector. Even so, returning to a home village poses the prospect of either dilution of wealth or social censure. Thus the new possibilities for establishing personal financial assets are somewhat misaligned with traditions fostering redistribution of food and material wealth. Adolescent girls navigating the present social landscape get little guidance from traditional social norms. Meanwhile, many of them have parents with little experience with wage-earning jobs and, as a result, they lack the information or experience to advise them.

Public commentary on weight—thin or fat, losing or gaining—is routine in Fiji and is also commonly experienced. For example, only approximately a quarter of school-going adolescent girls in the aforementioned 2007 study have *never* heard they are "too big" from either their family or their friends. Moreover, more than a quarter hear this sentiment often, almost all, or all the time from family members; peers give this message frequently (22 percent) as well. Young women critique themselves as "too big" with alarming frequency, with two-thirds of a representative sample endorsing this self-appraisal at least sometimes. Taken together, critiques of fatness—from family, peers, and one-self—are now normative in Fiji; these findings reflect a reversal from previous approbation of large size and are oddly paradoxical with the vigorous and persistent defense of robust appetite, evidenced in routine administration of indigenous medicines to prevent and treat macake.

The known adverse impact of weight-related teasing demonstrated in Western contexts raises concerns regarding the effects of critical weight commentary in Fiji. We examined the relation between these weight-related comments from peers and family on depressive symptoms (in the aforementioned 2007 school-based study and as measured by a dimensional CES-D score [Radloff 1977], a proxy indicator that has been locally validated in this study population; Opoliner et al. 2013). In a multivariate model, examining the relation between peer and family critical commentary on being "too big" and dysphoric affect (while adjusting for body mass index [BMI] and self-appraisal of being too big), peer commentary was significantly associated with depressive symptoms ($p = .003$), underscoring that such commentary may, indeed, not be entirely benign. By contrast, similar comments by family members were not independently associated with depressive symptoms. A plausible explanation for this discrepancy is that weight management is expected and therefore socially acceptable and tolerable from parents. Indeed, family commentary about being "too large" or "too fat" may actually be interpreted as positive feedback in some instances. A similar contrast was identified when we examined peer and family critique of weight in a multivariate model adjusting for self-appraisal and BMI, in our finding that peer critique was associated with strength of desire to enhance social standing by weight control (p = .02), whereas family critique was not.

Another relevant and potentially worrisome finding is that the strength of desire to navigate up the social hierarchy through weight management is weakly, but significantly, correlated with depressive symptoms (r = .09; p = .04) and moderately and highly significantly correlated with global (overall) eating pathology (r = .27; p < .0001). Finally, a significant relationship was observed between the perceptions that one can improve social standing through weight management (specifically) and improve social standing (generally) among the highest weight young women in the study, whereas this association was only marginally statistically significant among the lowest weight women.

Additional seemingly paradoxical findings support the ambiguity of social norms concerning appetite, consumption, and fatness over the past decade in Fiji. This ambiguity was especially apparent during interviews with underweight young women identified by weight and height measurement in our study. Following our study protocol, we invited respondents with a body mass index < 17.5 kg/m² for a diagnostic interview to evaluate whether or not they might have anorexia nervosa and benefit from assistance in accessing health care. In contrast to a blanket endorsement of thinness in admiration of television characters that had been evident in the context of interviews conducted almost a decade earlier (Becker 2004; Becker et al. 2002), several of the respondents denied concern about gaining *some* weight (which would be inconsistent with the fear of weight gain even while too thin that typifies anorexia nervosa) while also expressing concern about gaining too much weight or becoming too fat (*levulevu hivisia*). Notably, responses were contextualized against perceived social norms and family expectations that would situate them between the two extremes of being either too thin or too fat. Instead, a number of these young women articulated a weight goal of being "just right" (*varausia ga*) (Becker and Thomas 2015). This middle ground is interesting both in its contrast with the

(American) desire to be thin and thinner that characterizes anorexia nervosa, but also in its rationalization as avoiding pitfalls of social censure for being either too thin to be strong or too large to move well. Both extremes represented a body habitus likely to undermine contributions to community and household. This desire to conform to community standards of capacity to contribute is quite consistent with strong valuation of the state of being "grown well," or jubu vina, as markers of strength and vitality, which are essential to community integration. This anchoring of weight goals to the social center also contrasts with a desire for exceptionalism (as might be reflected in an extremely thin body) familiar in other cultural contexts where obesity is unequivocally stigmatized.

These findings placed the frequently concurrent use of both appetite stimulants and herbal purgatives in a new light. Whereas both are tied to use of the indigenous pharmacopoeia, and the purgatives could possibly have been a means of mitigating appetite, the concurrent use of medicine to preempt macake and herbal purgatives (or purging by other means) is also consistent with a desire to achieve conformity with respect to body size: a weight that is not exceptional, but rather "just enough." In this respect, these young women can avoid social censure for the stigma attached to either fatness or thinness. Stigmatization of thinness—even at the same time as it is valorized in locally available media—is manifest in the distaste reflected in an insult referencing thinness (*lila*) and as well as vigorous critique of families that fail to feed and care for their children properly. Weight loss in a child, for example, is read as either disease or social neglect or incompetence (Becker 1994). Although Fijians understand the indigenous illness macake to be prevalent and treatable, sufficient concern exists to encourage routine prophylactic dosing of herbal medications that are effective in managing it. In the context of community vigilance for weight changes, weight and its management are located in social space. For this reason, it should not surprise that weight loss similarly could be co-managed between mother and daughter. Although we were aware of respondents using indigenous purgatives "off label," we also heard stories about mothers (and other adult family members) procuring purgatives for their daughters. For example, one young woman who had received a purgative from her aunt discussed the responsibility of a family to manage weight:

> They like, they talk about her family, what are her parents doing or what do they think about what she's doing. Some of the girls they don't eat a lot, like me, but they used to go fat. Some of them they are really fatter than me.

But they, they used to say, what are their parents doing? They don't even care about her. . . . And they have to try and solve her problems. (I-23)

Whereas the concurrent use of these two weight-management strategies might be regarded as benign titration of two familiar remedies in the indigenous pharmacopoeia, our findings also showed that young women whose eating symptoms were primarily characterized by herbal purgative use (the "herbal purgative class") had significantly greater eating pathology than nonpurging women. Moreover, this herbal purgative class had significantly greater eating disorder–related distress and impairment than young women in the "bulimia nervosa–like class," comprising respondents who reported self-induced vomiting and a high frequency of binging, among other related symptoms (Thomas et al. 2011).

DECODING THE COMPLEXITY OF BODY IDEALS IN FIJI

The recent history of migrating body-weight ideals in Fiji might have opaque antecedents in many ways but inarguably establishes body-size ideals as plastic, fluid, and polyvalent. There are remarkable similarities with the trajectory of body-shape ideals and the emerging stigmatization of fatness elsewhere on the globe, but there are also striking dissimilarities. Much of this emerging story is evident in the course of flexible ideas, not just about ideal body size, but also in the new space for pursuing social aspirations through weight management.

Notwithstanding the parallels to the pursuit of thinness as a body ideal in late twentieth-century mainstream American culture, local models for the mechanics of weight management and its relation to upward social mobility warrant close scrutiny for their differences. These include the relation of dietary patterns with social and physical health, the bidirectionality of physical activity and weight, and the uncertain relation among weight, flexibility, and social mobility. The quantitative data presented here are just one proxy for the complex and dynamic relations among diet, weight, social norms, and upward social mobility in contemporary Fiji. These relations are also discernible in the contours of a metastory about body ideals, social standing, and rapid economic development in Fiji in which the *polyvalence* of weight and social standing is considered or exploited for social navigation. The interesting inflection point in Fiji relates not just to how ideals change but to how ideals migrate from being the object of admiration to the object of aspiration. Authority and responsibility for cultivation of body shape and weight traditionally were attributed not to an individual but to his or her family and community. Despite these changes, evidence demonstrates that aspirational and pragmatic work around body-weight management is still located in social space and may also be pursued as a joint project. In this and in many other ways (such as in spirit possession and certain kinds of illness episodes), bodies in Fiji can be understood to index social connection and social harmony, rather than solely personal characteristics. Elsewhere, such as in the United States, bodies serve as compelling vehicles for achievement. Whatever core values bodies encode and display in weight and size, they are conceived of as self-managed in this context. The prestige associated with thinness is premised on the value (and scarcity) of self-restraint and dogged adherence to a fitness routine. Much relies on the presumption of self-agency in careful stewardship of appetite and weight. Injudicious stewardship of appetite, diet, and physical activity likewise is read into the fat body.

As noted above, fat stigma surely is informed by lay understandings of the (patho)genesis of obesity, which often locate responsibility for the regulation of appetite and weight with individuals. This understanding persists even in the setting of alternate etiologic models—for example, energy imbalance relating to dietary quality and physical activity constrained by social structural barriers and heritable set points. In Fiji, however, there is a positive interpretation of robust weight as well as negative valence that attaches to low weights. The plurality of etiologies may suggest that a middle-ground weight, *varausia ga*, is deemed a safe and brilliant hedge. The symbolic import of size commentary tilts toward an appraisal of capacity to labor that somewhat defies strategic calibration: too thin and they are weak, even possibly self-absorbed; too large and their mass slows them, disadvantaging their domestic work. Too much thinness or fatness is perceived to jeopardize the highly socially valued capacity to contribute to family and community needs in Fiji. Likewise, either may be read as the legacy of social neglect and poor co-management of weight. The ceremonial obligations to engage in reciprocal caregiving and consumption are dissonant not only with social disapproval of obesity in Fiji but also with pragmatic exigencies of navigating rapidly changing economic opportunities. In this respect, the outsize proportion of respondents our study found who affirmed purging or purgative use may relate not to an unmitigated passion to achieve thinness but to an attempt to avoid the double bind inherent in conforming to traditions that no longer fit with economic realities. As Fijian adolescents survey the reconfigured landscape of economic opportunity and social norms they are mindful too of the penalty of stigma that attaches to body size—whether thin or fat—that tells a story of social alienation.

NOTES

1. The Fijian population described in this chapter is the iTaukei—formerly termed "ethnic"—Fijian population. This indigenous ethnic group comprises approximately half of Fiji's total population.

2. In the interview excerpts, S denotes the study participant and I denotes the interviewer. The study participant ID number is included to indicate which comments are from the same or different respondents.

CHAPTER EIGHT

Glocalizing Beauty

Weight and Body Image in the New Middle East

SARAH TRAINER

I sit in a coffee shop on a college campus with three sophomores, all women. Chatting with me—the adult who is not a professor but who spends time talking to students about health, lifestyle, and local culture—gives them something new to do. The young women talk about "girls they know who count calories too much" and "girls who are too thin," as well as the difference between families in which everyone is naturally thin and families in which everyone tries to be thin. They debate whether genetics or lifestyle contribute more to weight trajectories.

From there, one of the women segues into a discussion of the upcoming International Film Festival. Last year she volunteered and became stuck in a mob of screaming female fans when an international film star arrived. Never again, she says. Another starts texting without looking at her phone; she says she texts in class all the time without being caught—and that she has to multitask to stay awake in some lectures. The subject reminds her that she is due for a Red Bull. She then picks up her friend's copy of Hello! *magazine and points out the latest gossip about the Kardashians, in particular, the plastic surgery Kim Kardashian may have had on her face, breasts, waist, thighs, and so forth.*

—SARAH TRAINER, field notes, January 2011

The in-English conversation cited above shows no local rootedness. It was a conversation that could have occurred on any college campus anywhere in the modern world, and it highlights the globalizing influences that touch young women's lives, ranging from international media (*Hello!*) to transnational products (Red Bull) to beauty and body concerns.

In reality, the conversation also included all sorts of local specificities. For example, Arabic words and phrases were sprinkled throughout, the three students could not leave their campus without parental or administrative approval, and the women all wore their "national dress" of a black *abaya* (overgarment) and *shayla* (hijab/headscarf/veil). The nuances and context of this conversation thus helped root it in a specific time and place: the city of Dubai in the United Arab Emirates (UAE) in early 2011. My companions were young, local Emirati women attending public university within the UAE. The constant juxtaposition of local with global, as well as traditional with modern, dominates these young women's lives. And nowhere are these contradictions more evident than in discussions about obesity, weight, and body ideals.

Young Emirati women in the UAE of today sit at a nexus between local "tradition," albeit a reimagined and glamorized "Emirati tradition" (Bristol-Rhys 2010; Davidson 2009, 2008), and globalized, "modern" progress. For them, perceptions of beauty are increasingly "glocalized"—shaped both by the unique culture and context of their home as well as the rapidly accelerating influence of attitudes and behaviors common in more modern, Westernized areas. They must navigate new social and biological realities that include explosive national development and rising rates of obesity within the country. They also face a recent proliferation of public health and media-driven messages that underscore the idea that obesity is a negative condition (Brewis 2014, 2011; Goffman 1963; Granberg et al. 2008; Greenhaulgh and Carney 2014; Ogden and Clementi 2010) and that they should strive for the ideal of a thin body. At the same time, they are embedded in local communities that emphasize family ties, group affiliations, and key rules and expectations of behavior among young women (Bristol-Rhys 2010; Al-Sharekh 2007). As a result, women continually negotiate disparate expectations with respect to how they look. Appearance profoundly affects their navigation of professional, social, and familial spaces, as does the ever-changing and circumstance-specific priority given to traditional versus modern demands. In this context, the likelihood of their miscalculation is extremely high, a fact that provokes considerable stress and anxiety.

Between 2009 and 2011, I conducted ethnographic research in the UAE, a tiny federation of seven states (emirates) located in the southern Arabian Peninsula in the Middle East. This longitudinal study was based on extensive semistructured and unstructured interviewing and the collection of anthropometric data from just over one hundred female students attending two different public universities within the country. One institution was a commuter university and was located in the emirate of Dubai, and the other included dormitories for the students and was located in the emirate of Abu Dhabi. These participant-driven data were contextualized with my own extensive participant observation throughout the public spaces and university campuses of the seven emirates of the UAE.

As a result of a remarkably rapid development trajectory over the past half a century—fueled, quite literally, by the discovery and then systematic exploitation of its oil fields—the UAE has experienced an "obesity epidemic" in recent years, with well-documented increases in obesity, overweight, and associated chronic diseases at the national level (HAAD 2013; WHO 2014b, 2014c, 2014d, 2014e, 2014f; WHO-EMRO 2014a, 2014b, 2003). Globalization and modernization have brought consumer products, transnational retail companies, processed foods, labor-saving devices, and urbanization: all of the factors commonly cited to explain rising rates of obesity globally (Popkin 2009; WHO 2014e; WHO-EMRO 2003). These processes also have increased local exposure, especially among young people, to ideas about health and body through the education system, public health infrastructure, and transnational media. One result of these developments is that even as obesity has increased at the national level, so too has the idealization of thin bodies and a tendency to stigmatize fat bodies.

In an environment marked by material wealth, in a country where official public health statistics document dramatic recent increases in obesity among Emirati women over thirty years of age, extremely low body weights and body fat percentages were extremely common in my sample of female university students (see Trainer 2012 for an extended discussion).[1] An accompanying statistical analysis demonstrated that factors such as socioeconomic status, marital status, and even dietary quality (based on twenty-four-hour food recalls) were not good predictors of weight among these young women. In this case, the "homogenizing forces" of universal and free access to state-sponsored benefits such as health care and education smoothed out socioeconomic differences with respect to weight, particularly in terms of increasing women's knowledge of and access to weight-management strategies. Exposure to media messages that equate thinness with health and attractiveness was almost universal in this cohort. Concern over weight and "being fat," direct engagement with weight-loss strategies and other methods of bodily self-discipline (including exercise and the adoption of girdle-like clothing such as Spanx), and the casual equating of a "fat" individual body with laziness and even backwardness were common among the students in this study. Moreover, these trends are widespread. Almost three-quarters of young Emirati women currently attend institutions of higher education (Kemp 2013; UAE Government 2014; UAE Ministry of

Education 2014; UAE Ministry of State 2008; UN and League 2013). As a result, they must engage actively with dramatically different notions of beauty and weight ideals—as well as bodily practices—than the generations before them did.

Western notions tying together self, identity, and personal morality at the site of the individual body have become increasingly popular frameworks worldwide. The preoccupation with bodily self-discipline through the denial of food, and the ways in which this preoccupation reflects ingrained ideas about self-worth, has deep roots in the West, especially for women (Becker 1995; Brewis, Hruschka, and Wutich 2011; Counihan 1999; Gimlin 2002; Lester 1997; Ogden and Clementi 2010). The emphasis on bodily thinness as both an ideal and an ongoing project of work, however, gathered momentum in the West over the course of the last century. Partly, this increased focus on "body projects" occurred in reaction to greater global food stability and the increasingly transnational beauty industry's activities (Becker 1995; Brown and Konner 1987; Brumberg 1988; Reischer and Koo 2004; Miller 2006).

In this context, it is striking to observe similar attitudes and projects reflected in the discourses and activities of local women living in the Arab Gulf today. Even as recently as twenty years ago, the UAE (and neighboring countries) still had sharply different ideas about beauty, body, self-discipline, and body-based social capital compared to those that dominated in the West. This is no longer the case. Nevertheless, local culture continues to form a subtext to many conversations about women's bodies and "family" and "tradition" retain power, both as ideological frameworks and in day-to-day practice. In this respect, the notions of a solo project of self-improvement via weight loss or of a woman possessing individual "capital" based on achieving the desired thin body shape do not capture the reality of women's lives in the UAE (see Edmonds and Mears in this volume for an extended discussion of social and erotic capital). In the UAE, individual bodies continue to be reflections of—and, in turn, reflect upon—the families from which they originate.

"THE TRADITION" AND FEMALE BEAUTY

*The tradition was that a woman should have white skin
and long black hair and be heavy, with lots of curves.*
—SAMIA

Before, fat was considered exquisite in women.

—SALMA

The traditional idea of what looks good was a girl who "filled out her skin" because it showed her family had enough to feed her well . . . [which is why] my grandmother always tries to feed me.

—AMANI

All of the participants in this study agreed that when their grandmothers and grandfathers were young, when actual obesity in the UAE was far less of a problem than food scarcity (Heard-Bey 2004), a beautiful local woman was supposed to be "heavy" or "plump."[2] This somewhat vague category left open just what constituted heavy and plump, although participants were firm that this description applied to people much fatter than the current body ideal. Such narratives echo those documented by anthropologists working in other societies around the world, many of which could be characterized until very recently as "fat-positive" or, perhaps more properly, as exhibiting a preference for "bodily abundance" in women (Popenoe 2005). The appeal of female plumpness has been shown to be well established in the Middle East until well into the latter part of the twentieth century (e.g., Fernea 1965; Ghannam 1997). Globally, it has been documented in communities ranging from the Arabs of Niger (Popenoe 2004) to Fiji (Becker 1995) to Jamaica (Anderson-Fye et al., this volume; Sobo 1993).

Many young women noted that fat-positive attitudes still dominate their grandparents' thinking but resonate unevenly with their parents. Some mothers and fathers emphasized that women needed "more meat on their bones" (to quote Salma again), but other parents actively pushed their daughters to lose weight. Anthropologists in diverse societies around the world have documented comparable shifts in thinking about beauty and body, as well as the coexistence of old and new ideals among different cohorts experiencing profound socioeconomic change (Anderson-Fye et al., this volume; Anderson-Fye 2004; Brewis, Hruschka, and Wutich 2011).

Anthropological research (Popenoe 2004; Becker, this volume; Becker 1995) indicates that in many social contexts, bodies are considered profoundly communal in nature. A body project is conceived not as an individual project—affecting only how the individual body is perceived—but instead as a familial and/or community project. A body can serve as a status marker (for good or ill) for an entire family. This perspective stands in marked contrast to Western perceptions of the individual body, the individual body project, and individual work (such as weight loss) upon the body (Becker 1995; Bordo 1993; Feather-stone 1982; Giddons 1993; Turner 1984, 1982).

Body shape, appearance, weight, and adornment are increasingly viewed globally through a lens that ascribes individual responsibility and agency for said shape. This lens also views personal improvement projects at the site of the physical body as indicative of personal moral worth (Becker 1995; Dickins et al. 2011; Farrell 2011; Gimlin 2007, 2002; Greenhaulgh and Carney 2014; Ogden and Clementi 2010; Rothblum and Solovay 2009). Furthermore, experiences involving weight management, attitudes toward body image, social patterns affected by weight and beauty concerns, and deployment of body capital show gendered differences in many instances. Women disproportionately feel the impact of body and weight concerns (Becker 1995; Bordo 1993; Carpenter et al. 2000; Carryer 1997; Edmonds 2010; Edmonds and Mears, this volume; Gimlin 2007, 2002; Fallon 1990; Jackson 1992; Millman 1980; Nichter 2000; Orbach 1978; Rothblum and Solovay 2009; Wolf 1990).

Some of this thinking appears to have made inroads among local Emiratis in the UAE, most clearly demonstrated in frequent discussions that stigmatize larger bodies as "lazy" and "too fat." In other respects, however, female bodies remain communal projects in which family members still may interfere. The difference is that the projects now center more often on weight loss rather than the promotion of women who "fill out their skins."

Beauty and the Body in the Emirates
of the Twenty-First Century

One of the central points around which interviews tended to revolve related to the concept of the "ideal female body" in the UAE today, as well as perceived key elements of physical beauty. Participants expressed strong and diverse opinions on this subject, although the interviews reflected similar themes.

Public health and medical rhetoric in and about the UAE tends to portray obesity as not only common in the Emirati community but also normalized by it (Trainer 2013a). This attitude stands in direct contrast to the high level of awareness expressed by study participants regarding the medical risks of being overweight, as well as the significant social pressure they experienced to achieve a thin body. Participants universally agreed that most women in their age cohort desired a thin and toned body. This thin, toned body signals—to the local audience but also to a largely disembodied and imaginary Western gaze—an ability to meet modern expectations and demands. In other words, such a body is not a "failed" subject of modernization and overconsumption. Ideally, this modern body is clothed respectably in some version of the shayla and abaya, which in recent decades have solidified as key, visible markers of group belonging and (reimagined) local tradition for Emirati women (Bristol-Rhys 2010; Al Qasimi 2010; Trainer 2013b).

Research in the industrialized West (e.g., Greenhaulgh and Carney 2014; Grønning, Scambler, and Tjora 2013; Lunner et al. 2000; Ogden and Clementi 2010; Puhl and Heuer 2010, 2009; Thomas et al. 2008) indicates that obesity is highly stigmatized on an everyday basis, not only in terms of presumed lowered physical attractiveness but also in terms of assumed associated moral deficiencies, that is, laziness, messiness, and so on. Poor treatment related to obesity stigma and weight-based discrimination results in daily indignities and suffering across all manner of public and private spaces (Brewis 2014, 2011; Gimlin 2002; Hebl and Mannix 2003; Puhl and Heuer 2010, 2009). Reasons for such cultural biases include deeply ingrained cultural norms that portray weight gain as personal failure (Brewis 2014, 2011; Gimlin 2002; Maddox, Back, and Liederman 1968; Rogge 2004; Rothblum 1992; Stafford and Scott 1986), the increasing centrality of the physical body in the construction of social identities (Becker 1995; Bordo 1993), and the inability to hide or "mask" a large body (Boero 2012; Jones et al. 1984).

My study participants articulated a similar moral attitude, with most of the young women describing overweight and obese friends and family members as "lazy" or having "given up" on their health and appearance. Participants frequently characterized Emiratis as preferring to sit around talking, especially about food. One participant, Afra, said, "After my family eats lunch, we sit around, *yanni*, and discuss what to have for dinner!" Another participant, Fatimah, told me, "Fat people never do as well [on exams or at work] because their nutrition is bad." Here Fatimah extends negative connotations of obesity beyond laziness, basing her claim of poor performance in an alleged biological difference in terms of poor health and nutrition.

These characterizations proved particularly interesting when juxtaposed with the almost universal dissatisfaction participants expressed regarding their own bodies. Fatimah herself was "fat" according to biomedical categories and her own estimations—and she was extremely unhappy and self-conscious about her appearance. Similarly, Raniyah, told me, "I know I'm fat and that I need to make a diet." Sameera said in her first interview, "I will tell you the honest truth, Ms. Sara—I am thinking about my weight every second of every day, even when I'm studying or doing other things. . . . It is like a stone in my heart." Sameera had been to numerous doctors in her frantic efforts to lose weight, had been told repeatedly that she was morbidly obese, but had never been able to lose weight as directed or to come to terms with her "otherwise healthy" body. Two other participants mentioned that they had been identified as the "Fat One" in their respective social groups and as morbidly obese by their doctors. Both of them reported experiencing teasing at school and at home with respect to their weight.

Even participants who did not identify as "fat" expressed body dissatisfaction, saying they needed to lose weight, either overall or (more frequently) in their thighs and belly. Lara said in her first interview, "I hate my belly and want it to be more toned and my biceps are too big." She changed her exercise pattern over the time I knew her, from playing team sports at her university to attending classes at a ladies-only Fitness First; as a result, she lost weight over the course of my interviews with her. Sara told me, "I want a sexy body." When asked what this term meant to her, she said it involved losing her belly fat and being thinner through her waist and back. Indeed, the women articulated a ubiquitous refrain of being "slender" or "fit" in the waist and arms and thighs.

Participants often perceived themselves as "fat" overall or "fat" in problem areas. But although they equated obesity in *others* with ill health and laziness, they did not did not judge themselves as lazy or sick. Participants portrayed themselves as "knowing what was proper" (to quote Raniyah again), and as wanting to maintain the "proper" actions needed shrink their bodies. Their failures to do so represented "struggling," rather than "laz[iness]."

Some of the women who were overweight or obese (WHO 2014a) said they had always been bigger, even as children, and they blamed their difficulties losing weight on uncooperative genetics. Others adopted the opposite tactic and detailed ways in which they had been thinner as children and/or successfully (if temporarily) lost weight in the past. Some of the more nutritionally informed women whose measurements placed them in an overweight or obese category (WHO 2014a) added the corollary that even though they were larger, they had healthy lifestyles. Fatimah, for example, spent half an hour describing her "plant-based" diet and how nutritionally sound it was. Dana said she was frustrated because "I exercise more than lots of skinny girls I know, but I have big bones and a slow metabolism."

An even more widespread trend among the participants who expressed reservations about their existing body shape was a tendency to blame their inability to shrink their size on the stressful, busy schedules that they endured as university students. Many said that their schedules were so busy that they sacrificed health as a result. Amani voiced a common complaint when she said that she joined a gym "and for the first month I went two to four times a week, but these past weeks I haven't done anything because I've been busy with classes and projects." Participants thus preserved a sense of moral superiority vis-à-vis other Emiratis, not through different behaviors, or even based on an assumption that their physical bodies adhered more closely to the thin ideal, but via different explanations and rhetoric about the reasons producing particular bodies that did not conform. Taylor's research (2006) among adolescents in the United States shows a similar gap between the American teenagers' stigmatizing comments about the alleged moral sloppiness associated with *other* large bodies and their tendency to sidestep personal moral responsibility when discussing their *own* bodies.

Judgments of "laziness" among Emiratis often extended beyond notions of personal indulgence leading to weight gain and were deployed in both general critiques of modern UAE society and Emiratis. Western expatriates in the UAE, for example, often relied on stereotypes of wealthy, spoiled Emiratis. Such an attitude understandably offended many locals, but at the same time it was not infrequently mirrored in their own talk about themselves. Many participants were startled when I told them that the United States and many countries in Europe have very obese populations. They thought Westerners exercised more and ate more healthily than did locals. When asked whether Emiratis ever walk around outside, Lara responded, "Someone may see an ex-pat walking her dog but then the [Emirati] girl will still just tell her maid to walk her own dog." Nisa commented, "It's not that difficult to join a gym—but lots of [local] ladies don't bother. And [those that do] don't do it correctly—they go and spend the whole time talking or on their computers while foreign ladies exercise." Similarly, Dana said that many girls at her university "don't know how to exercise properly—lots of them wear flip-flops or other inappropriate shoes; some of them wear the wrong clothes, leaving their abayas on and just hiking them up. . . . And one day I was at the gym and a girl came up and said, 'Do you mind me asking why you're drinking water when you're exercising? Because you'll lose more weight if you don't drink water.'" Many participants who made such comments went on to make equally pessimistic comments about Emiratis' performances and competence (or lack thereof) in the workplace and classroom. They couched these comments in terms of certain "other" Emiratis not knowing how to work, exercise, or eat healthily, compared to themselves. At the same time, the women also talked about these issues in terms of concern for "us," "our country," and "our people." In this sense, they contrasted everyday realities (framed as "failed" local attempts to successfully modernize) with an imagined ideal in which they were able to balance modern and traditional demands.

The sense of moral high ground that participants articulated did not focus only on "fat, lazy" Emiratis but also on the women they saw as "too thin" and obsessed with their appearance. When I asked what an ideal body looked like, every participant echoed Samia's description: "Not too fat, not too thin . . . a small waist but with curves . . . yanni, normal." Participants repeatedly used the word *normal* and then contrasted this assessment with girls on campus who "took it too far," became "too skinny, like sticks," and were "obsessed with fashion." Lara used these phrases, but many other women echoed them. "I want to be the right weight for my body, nothing extreme," Layla told me. Many cited friends and family members who lost too much weight and looked ill in consequence, plus "skeletal" models and celebrities, as examples they did not want to emulate. Women therefore appear to walk a fine line between (1) failing to modernize via the possession of a fat body that indiscriminately overconsumes and (2) becoming "too modern" and indiscriminately consumed with a vain preoccupation over appearance, body, and extreme weight-loss and beauty projects.

How do we reconcile rhetoric about a "normal body" being best with near-constant dissatisfaction participants and their friends expressed verbally and/ or behaviorally (via dieting)? One contributing factor to this apparent contradiction emerged. I asked participants to identify someone (known to us both) who was "normal" and embodied their beauty ideal. In response, participants overwhelmingly cited Kim Kardashian as possessing a beautiful body. Beyoncé was the second most popular choice. Stars of this ilk describe working out multiple hours a day, five to six days a week, and "watching what they eat" (i.e., they indulge in drastic dieting), and they are rumored to have had plastic surgery. They are not easily (or inexpensively) emulated.

"Normal" in this instance actually references a toned, hourglass-shaped body. In this context, critiques of Emirati girls who were "too thin" were as devastating for some participants as the critiques of girls who were "too fat." Weight-related teasing could be vicious and targeted both obese and underweight women. Several participants whose measurements placed them in the underweight category (WHO 2014a) expressed considerable frustration because they were naturally too thin, could not gain weight, and therefore bore the brunt of teasing from other female students. Reema, for example, who was drastically underweight, told me her weight and frame had been a continual source of unhappiness for her since her arrival at university: "My friends . . . always tell me I'm too skinny and get really mean about it and I think about my weight all the time now." I asked, "But don't they all want to be thin themselves?" She answered: "They all want to be thinner, but not as thin as me—they want to be normal but thin."

The magazines students read—*Hello!* and *Ahlan* were popular—reinforced transnational messages about beauty and glamour, showing a parade of beautiful, thin women in beautiful, expensive dresses. The television channel Dubai One aired a mix of American and British movies, as well as local advertisements and news segments that featured beautiful, thin Emirati women. Similar images were available on channels showing Bollywood movies, Australian and Korean soap operas, and the Lebanese equivalent of MTV. At the same time, UAE public health messages focused on the "obesity epidemic" and the importance of weight loss: several "health and beauty" fairs held on the university campuses also focused on weight loss (including through products like diet pills, aloe vera drinks, and cellulite creams) and beauty regimes (skin-care and hair products, makeup, etc.).

Participants universally agreed that exposure to Western media shaped younger generations of Emiratis' beauty ideals. Becker's later work (Becker et al. 2011; Becker, this volume) in Fiji among young Fijian women provides useful insight into this pattern, for this research showed a pronounced correlation between the extent of transnational media exposure within a social network and the degree to which young women within that social network exhibited new ideals about thin bodies and dieting strategies. In the UAE, women were quite critical of the influence of Western media in the abstract and ambivalent toward it in terms of daily practice and attitudes. Although several participants disapproved of the politics and foreign policies of the United States (as well as the lifestyles showcased in *Keeping up with the Kardashians*), those sentiments did not reduce the influence of the American entertainment industry's body ideals, nor the myth that Westerners practice healthier habits of eating and exercise.

I observed advertisements and products from US, European, and Asian companies selling cosmetics, skin-care regimes, and diet products everywhere in the UAE during the course of fieldwork. Peiss (2002) presents a compelling story of the activities of American cosmetics companies abroad in the decades since World War II, arguing that Americans have systematically "exported now ubiquitous images of glamorized, sexualized female beauty . . . for over seven decades" (101). In this regard, Kaufman and Nichter's discussion of consumer culture as a "culture of mass consumption" (2012, 117) also is relevant here. They argue that participants in such cultures buy and use transnational products to emulate the lifestyles shown in global product advertisements. Although some participants described this influence as part of the alleged moral decline of the UAE, they nonetheless wanted to look like certain American stars. They expressed this desire even as they acknowledged that the representations they saw were skewed. In other words, the women knew these advertisements and programs pushed them toward specific ideals and images. Both Nisa and Lara used the same phrase — "they [the female university students] are not stupid" — when talking about skewed advertising.

These young women in the UAE are not alone in their frustrated awareness of their own attempts to comply with near-impossible norms. Medical anthropologists and feminist scholars (Bordo 1993; Diamond and Quinby 1988; Kaw 1993; Lee 2009; McLaren 2002; Orbach 1978; Rothblum and Solovay 2009; Shildrick and Price 1998; Wolf 1990) have written extensively on this subject, including examining the ways in which dieting, plastic surgery, cosmetics, and other efforts combine to create highly gendered bodily practices and forms of discipline. Foucault (1977, 1973) established the foundation for much of this research with his work on discipline at the site of the body. Foucault's theories with respect to discipline in modern societies stress that it is both externally and internally imposed as a result of the creation of certain norms and expected adherence to these norms. Individuals may realize they are subjecting themselves to self-discipline to adhere to a collectively imagined norm, but that knowledge does not lessen the power of that norm. In the UAE, that norm relies heavily on relatively recent images from the United States, Europe, and Bollywood. Nevertheless, their influence on attitudes and ideals has been enormous over the course of just two generations.

Even so, the UAE is not a modern state inasmuch as power still flows through networks based on family, tribe, ethnicity, and patronage (Trainer 2013b). Individual advancement (or lack thereof) is embedded in these larger networks and forward progress (or lack thereof) reflects these power distributions. Emirati women face many contradictions as modern and traditional expectations and pressures flow simultaneously through their daily lives. The importance they give those respective expectations shifts as they navigate different spaces and audiences, different social patterns and norms, and different rules of social engagement (Bourdieu 1990, 1984). Much has been written about the contradictory demands facing Arab women across many different national and cultural contexts (El-Guindi 1999; Hasso 2011; Abu-Lughod 1993; Mahmood 2005; Sobh, Belk, and Gressel 2014; Al-Sharekh 2007; Al-Sharekh and Springborg 2008), where the simultaneous expectation is that the women perform modernity and tradition, in their education and career trajectories, in their home, and in their dress and general comportment. The "not too thin, not too fat . . . small waist . . . curves" admonition straddles this line as well, and its very vagueness can add to the stress that woman feel.

Weight—and the physical body itself—is an interesting lens with which to view this struggle, as ethnographic evidence from other regions demonstrates. For example, Talukdar (2012) discusses the often opposing forces buffeting middle- and upper-class Indian women living in urban India today with respect to image and weight, as well as the ways in which these index larger conflicts. Talukdar's own ethnographic findings showed the Indian women in her study negotiated local cultural expectations of what a "good" Indian woman looks like vis-à-vis the effects globalization and modernization in India have had on the female body. She detailed how these women juggled concern with their appearance and weight loss with worries that they might appear vain or self-centered if they lost too much weight. In addition, they had to navigate competing definitions of an ideal body. Anderson-Fye (2004) highlighted similar competing ideals about what women's bodies should look like and weigh in an island community in Belize. This work explored the ways these ideals affected the young women in the community specifically, as well as their more general impact on the attitudes of locals and foreign tourists.

Negotiating Body Projects with Family

Within the larger sociocultural environment created by media and medical messages, UAE participants noted their peers and families had a profound impact
on their attitudes and behaviors. Traditionally, in the region, the extended
family unit was the essential socioeconomic unit, especially for women; one of
the current points of fracture for many Emiratis is the contradiction between
the continuing moral obligation still associated with putting one's family first
and the fact that more social and work opportunities with nonfamily members are now available (Bristol-Rhys 2010; Crabtree 2007; Al-Sharekh 2007;
Al-Sharekh and Springborg 2008). This conflict echoes Talukdar's argument
that "women with access to modern worlds but who are nevertheless expected
to satisfy traditional definitions of feminine propriety, create 'in-between'
rationales to partake in both worlds" (2012, 4). Such rationales are attempts to
reconcile seemingly oppositional expectations with respect to women's bodily
practices.

This conflict offered relevant background for my own fieldwork since all of
the unmarried participants at the commuter university at which I studied lived
at home and all of the unmarried participants at the university with dormitories
went home every weekend. Thus much of the women's off-campus socializing
centered on their families. This meant that many of the anecdotes that participants shared involved a cousin, sibling, parent, or aunt/uncle. For example, "My
aunts are fat and have diabetes but my father [their brother] is more careful"
and "My cousin's children eat junk food all the time but my sister won't let her
daughter drink soda." Several participants mentioned that their mothers and/
or fathers harassed them to lose weight, and others cited teasing from siblings
or cousins. Both male cousins and brothers participated in teasing: one participant told me her father and brothers called her Humpty Dumpty in high school,
and another said that her brother recently brought all of his exercise equipment
into her room and told her that she should use it. These male family members
also discussed what they wanted their wives to look like in front of participants.
Such comments sometimes aggravated the women. Lila told me, "My brothers
are not so tall and one is losing his hair on top . . . but they still want to marry a
beautiful woman and talk about what 'beautiful' means all the time," and Sara
said, "I have to hear about what a beautiful woman is all the time because my
brother wants to get married and talks and talks about it." On the other hand,

participants did listen to and internalize these opinions, voiced by their male relatives, especially if they did not have access to other male perspectives.

Discussions about weight were also prominent in certain families. Some women portrayed their families as embarking on a group project to lose weight and improve their overall health. Shaikha, for example, said that she and her siblings kept a scale in their living room and weighed themselves on it regularly, in front of each other. Similarly, Nisa said that her whole family was interested in nutrition. When asked why, she answered that her brother had been obese when he was younger. When he turned fifteen, he joined a gym and began a diet. His choice led the entire family to join Fitness First, and since then they have all tried to be careful about portion sizes and "eliminating oil and salt." Nisa also talked constantly about weight-related issues with her mother and older sister; she said the conversations helped them feel closer to each other. During the first ten months of my study, Nisa and her sister embarked on a joint project to lose weight (although neither was in the overweight category) in time for the sister's wedding in May 2010.

This again bolsters the point that body ideals and rhetoric about personal responsibility have shifted dramatically in the UAE, but women's bodies are still viewed as familial projects—if not by the women themselves, then certainly by the families. Becker (this volume) makes a similar point in the context of Fiji. The notions of a solo project of self-improvement via weight loss, a person carrying fat stigma alone, and a woman possessing personal capital based on achieving the desired thin body shape do not capture the reality of women's lives in the UAE (see Edmonds and Mears, this volume; Hruschka, this volume). Individual bodies are inextricably embedded in the families from which they originate.

NEGOTIATING WEIGHT CONCERNS WITH FRIENDS

Despite the importance of family opinion and interactions, many women echoed Samia, who said, "Friends are more important [than family] in affecting girls' ideas about weight." Bodies and weight may be important family projects, but friends' opinions about what constitutes a beautiful body are considered more trustworthy in a globalized market. Given the rate of cultural change and the resulting discrepancies between generations in terms of lifestyles, skills, education, health, beauty aesthetics, and beauty regimes and technologies, reliance on peers in this realm seems a reasonable approach.

Since most participants' friendships were formed at university, the majority of the nonfamily social interactions cited involved other university students and took place on campus. This context (which was female dominated to begin with, given gender ratios at university), together with cultural strictures on casual socializing between the genders, meant that most peer socializing was all female. As noted previously, the study participants registered a widespread emphasis on being thin. All but a handful of the participants commented on this, and many added some negative corollary related to the all-female environments. Salma, for example, told me, "The all-girl environment [at the university] . . . is really hard on me—all of the peer pressure is toxic, with all the girls looking at each other and comparing weights." Zaynab added, "I look around [the central food court on campus] . . . and I see all these thin girls and think, 'Oh, I want to look like that!'"

Conversations about weight were everywhere on the campuses, and typically they were not positive. The discussions focused on women who were too fat (or sometimes too thin) and strategies for losing (or gaining) weight. Fatimah, for example, started her second interview remarking that after our first conversation, she had started to notice that everyone she knew, including friends and family, talked about weight a lot: "It comes up in every single conversation with my friends, my mother, and my mother's friends—they all want to talk about dieting, even when they're thin." Many of the participants reported that their circles of friends talked about their weight and body size often and perceived problems with both qualities. Samia said, "All my friends talk about being fat. . . . If someone says [that she is fat], then you must be supportive and tell her that losing weight might be a good idea." Zahra told me that, to tease each other, she and her friends at university say, "Hi, Fatty!" Many women reported being teased and even bullied by female peers on campus about their weight. Lara, irritated with her constantly dieting friends, said, "It's ridiculous when my super-super skinny friends tell me that I'm thinner than them. . . . I have love handles, who cares, but there they are, 'Look at my thighs!' and I'm like, 'What thighs, yanni?!'"

Some participants said conversations about weight and "being fat" were uncommon among their friends. They explained this relative anomaly by noting that their friends were not as consumed with appearance as other young women. Noor, for instance, said that her friends talk about weight "sometimes" but not as much as "the girls who worry so much about fashion." On the other hand, Latifah initially told me in the first interview that her friends did not often worry about weight, but she amended this opinion in her second interview. In this latter interview, she said that after she told them about joining my study, her friends all suddenly had a great deal to say about weight and wishing they could lose weight. Latifah concluded that many had been worrying privately about their bodies but had simply not felt comfortable raising the topic before she provided them with the conversational opening.

College women worrying aloud about weight constitutes an activity that could take place on virtually any university campus anywhere in the world today (Ousley, Cordero, and White 2008; Salk 2012; Taylor 2006). Since Nichter (2000) first coined the term *fat talk* to describe this phenomenon, researchers have has identified similar patterns across different educational contexts (Anderson-Fye et al., this volume; Ousley, Cordero, and White 2008; Payne et al. 2011; Salk 2012). Our own recent work on a US campus identified similar patterns in the use of the word *fat* to self-describe and use against others (Trainer et al. 2015a).

MEN, ROMANCE, AND WEIGHT

Did male peers play a significant role in women's conversations about weight and constructions of the ideal feminine body? Yes, to differing degrees. When it came to male friends, many participants either did not associate much with boys or else did not admit that they did. Of those that were willing to talk about male friends, Lara was vehement in saying that "men don't like super skinny girls!" But Habiba told me that based on what she heard from the boys that she knew, "guys don't want fat girls anymore—they tell their mothers, 'Find me a girl who is thin as a stick.'" When asked whether thin as a stick was the ideal, Habiba responded, "Well, *I* don't want to be that thin . . . but boys are silly." Two students, Aisha and Khadijah, offered additional details:

I: Do your friends talk about weight and "being fat" a lot?
AISHA: Oh, yes—a lot.
KHADIJAH: But Aisha is the worst. She's constantly talking about how she
   needs to lose weight.
[The conversation turns to a debate about Aisha's alleged weight obsession
   before I ask a new question.]
I: How do you know what boys look for?
AISHA: From our brothers.
KHADIJAH: And from friends who are boys.

I: How do you have male friends here?

AISHA: Well, from the Internet . . . especially Facebook. But we go to social gatherings with boys. . . .

I: But don't your parents mind?

KHADIJAH: We mostly tell them that we are going out with girlfriends. . . . Our parents are very traditional.

AISHA: I'm the youngest, my parents are old and don't care as much with me—my older sisters tired them already. If my father asks for more details [about where I'm going], I just tell him, "You really don't want to know" and he doesn't ask more. [Both laugh.]

I: So what do your male friends say about women's appearance?

AISHA: Emiratis can be very, um, blunt about how someone looks . . . [and] boys tell us if they think something [clothing or makeup] looks bad. But it would be really difficult if they ever said anything about weight.

KHADIJAH: We would be devastated. Worse than with girls. . . . [Apparently, none of their male friends have ever said anything really negative about their weight, however.]

AISHA: Yes. Emiratis can always tell if you are too chubby, even in an abaya—and they comment on it. But it's worse with no abaya because we wear tight jeans and clothes underneath.

KHADIJAH: Aisha gets very nervous before social gatherings where she has to take her abaya off.

AISHA: Tight jeans give me a, um, a muffin top [gestures toward her stomach]. Even my sister said so.

Highlighted here is the worry about weight that figures so prominently in their thinking and conversations. The account also illustrates the importance that the two women attach to comments male friends make about their appearance as well as to the male gaze in general (Taylor 2006).

The male gaze becomes far more pivotal when the issue of marriage arises.[3] Drastic socioeconomic and cultural changes in recent years have dramatically increased education and employment opportunities for women within the UAE (Kemp 2013; UAE 2014; UAE Ministry of Education 2014; UAE Ministry of State 2008; UN and League 2013). Nevertheless, participants emphasized that marriage is still considered of utmost importance for Emirati women. They also noted that local tradition, local interpretations of Islam, and (until very recently) citizenship laws that follow patrilineal lines conspire to make it disadvantageous for Emirati women to marry non-Emiratis. Such disadvantages did not apply, however, to Emirati men who married non-Emiratis. This imbalance makes the marriage market extremely competitive from a female Emirati point of view, and therefore, it is at this point that the concept of "body capital" (Bourdieu 1986; Edmonds and Mears, this volume; Hakim 2010; Hruschka, this volume; Martin and George 2006) in the context of family-driven weight-loss projects becomes particularly important. In this chapter, following Edmonds and Mears (this volume), "body capital" refers specifically to body-centered capital based in beauty, aesthetic, sexual, and erotic ideals. Bodies accumulate differing amounts of capital, depending on how well they meet current preferences and ideals. This affects a person's—and, in a country such as the UAE, a family's—capacity to achieve desired outcomes (Becker 1995; Reischer and Koo 2004). A fat female body in the modern UAE impedes marriage opportunities, according to participants, because Emirati men of their generation stigmatize fat to the same degree that women do.

Participants consistently portrayed weddings as pivotal events in women's weight-loss trajectories. Fatimah remarked that "most of the girls here lose weight for events like weddings," a comment that many other participants echoed. Amirah had a sister who married partway through my fieldwork and Amirah not only reported that her sister went on a severe diet for six months before the wedding but that she herself also tried to lose weight for it, via severe dieting. Likewise, Maryam, who was engaged during the school year in which I met her, told me that she had scheduled her wedding for July, so that she had a month "to get in shape" after school finished for the summer. According to Maha, "The big thing is to lose weight when you get engaged so that you look good in your wedding dress," and several other participants said something similar, telling me that the bride focuses on looking "perfect" that one night and then can gain weight thereafter (and usually does, they added, especially once she begins to have babies).

What consistently emerged in the interviews were similar weight-loss strategies centered on the wedding event but enacted for slightly different reasons. First and foremost, the bride to be typically embarked on an ambitious regime to lose weight for the wedding. Additionally, however, female guests, and especially female relatives of the bride or groom, also strategized to reduce their sizes in time for the wedding. Emirati weddings are massive community events and, as a result, serve as an important venue for unmarried girls to be looked over by nonrelatives. Fatimah, for example, said that she needed to lose weight for her cousin's wedding in three months' time, because she too wanted to get married. What is interesting about the wedding-as-marriage-market, however, is that Emirati weddings are also single sex: the men and women typically attend parties in separate locations (sometimes even on different days). Thus the people that the unmarried young women dress to impress are the female relatives of eligible Emirati men.

Also interesting are the ways in which male opinions, expressed by prospective and current fiancés, begin to appear in the women's discourses about their bodies. For instance, Nisa said that her sister felt that she had achieved "the perfect weight" by the betrothal and was trying to maintain that weight until the wedding, even though "my sister's fiancé told his sister to tell my sister" that she needed to gain a little weight. By contrast, Sameera told me that her cousin backed out of a marriage agreement with her because he thought she was "too fat," as did another man: "I was particularly shocked my cousin would do that to me, but he works out and has four-packs [abs] and he doesn't think much of me." She said that she worries that she is never going to get married because of her weight.

The few already-married women in my study also reported interactions with their husbands with respect to weight and appearance. Sara has actually worried more about her looks since her marriage than she had earlier. She mentioned that she had been raised "very traditionally" by her grandmother and "never waxed anything or colored my hair . . . and now I color my hair and wax everything and even wear short skirts under my abaya, which shocks my mother." She mentioned that she is also much more conscious about her body and wants to lose some waist fat that she doesn't like and so she tries to walk regularly with her mother-in-law. Moreover, she and her husband tried to diet together occasionally.

Sara talked about her husband in far more romantic terms than other married participants did about their spouses. Far more typical was Hanan, who had been married four years and had two children by the time she participated in this study. Hanan described strict weight-loss regimes that she had adhered to, both before her wedding "so that I would look good for that first impression," as well as after the birth of each of her children. She was also, however, quite pragmatic when talking about marriage, spouses, and ideals:

> Both my brothers always said they wanted to marry a girl who was tall,
> with long hair and pale skin but then they married girls who were short

and darker-skinned—and one even cut her hair off! Whatever you think of [in terms of] your ideal, it fades and you settle into reality. . . . Look at me—my husband is five centimeters shorter than me! I always pictured myself with a man who was taller and with muscles so I could cuddle against him, like in the movies . . . and who was well educated [her husband worked in the army and didn't finished high school]. I almost didn't sign the marriage documents, but then, well, I decided he was a good man—and it's still true, he is. . . . But I only wear heels when I'm on campus.

Hanan was working extraordinarily hard to achieve a thin, toned body, but her impulse to do so did not arise from a desire to impress her husband. Similarly, she actually dressed *up* when she was on campus, compared to when she was home. Once again, she was doing all of this for a female audience.

This account shows that stress about weight in college-aged women may peak around events like weddings, but it doesn't disappear afterward. It also demonstrates that satisfying the male gaze (Taylor 2006) is a factor in stress about weight, but it is certainly not the only, or even the most dominant, one. Romance plays a role in many of these self-projects, but is not foremost in importance on an everyday basis. The primary audience most of the female Emirati students encounter is female, the result of different layers of formal and informal gender segregation on and off campus. Nonetheless, weddings have a very significant impact on health and weight in that they—along with other community events—reinforce the short-term-gain orientation of most young women's dieting projects.

CONCLUSION

Worry and stress over weight, as well as expressed stigma about fat and obese bodies, dominated university campuses in the UAE. As mentioned at the outset, young Emirati women today sit at a nexus between local tradition and globalized, modern progress and must constantly walk both worlds, with their often-contradictory expectations and demands. This often-discordant pressure affected all of the women I spoke with, regardless of where they and their families fell on the socioeconomic or traditional spectrum. Women were expected to show through their bodily practices and appearance that they could be respectful of their families and Emirati tradition while also navigating modernity. Nutrition and long-term health were not important from this per-spective, for the focus was on a "thin-normal" body that reflected a woman's ability to manage appearance without being labeled vain and to consume with-out overconsuming.

The pressure many women felt to achieve an idealized thin-but-not-skinny body for aesthetic reasons, without an accompanying concern with health and nutrition, resulted in troubling behavioral patterns. Their lifestyles were largely inactive and diets were poor (based on the 24-Hour Food and Activity Recalls I collected). Only about a quarter of the sample expressed worry about develop-ing diabetes or another chronic disease, even though all of the women had close family members with diabetes and/or heart disease. Concern over and aware-ness about current micronutrient deficiencies, anemia, and insufficient muscle mass were even lower among participants, despite alarming reports from cam-pus athletic directors and school nurses with whom I spoke that indicated high rates of anemia, bone loss, and other deficiencies among college students. In this context, it seems vital to ask how to shift public focus in the UAE from a myopic concern with obesity and weight loss to a more holistic notion of health. Perhaps even more important, we must shift the public focus away from stories that feed into unflattering stereotypes of young Emirati women as shallow and consumed with appearance. Instead, we should try to address the many pres-sures, local and global, that these women face in their everyday lives.

NOTES

1. See Trainer et al. (2015b) for a critique of international health's overreliance on BMI categories. In this instance, however, the numbers tell an interesting story, particularly in terms of changes in BMIs across time within the UAE and in terms of the differences between the national average and my sample.

2. All names used throughout this chapter are pseudonyms.

3. Boyfriends are becoming more common in the UAE, but few participants admitted to having one. Thus, here romance equals current or potential marriage.

Fat Matters

Capital, Markets, and Morality

REBECCA J. LESTER AND EILEEN P. ANDERSON-FYE

Taken together, the chapters in this volume illuminate several key issues involving the social and economic aspects of individual and group attitudes toward fat. Across different historical and cultural contexts, bodies with more fat have signaled and contributed to disparate levels of appeal and status. Sometimes they have held a positive valuation, at other times a great deal of stigma, and at yet other times a simultaneous segmented valuation such as by gender or urban/rural status. In contrast to studies that take "the body" to be simply a material instantiation of cultural values, the chapters in this volume consider the body as both a product of social forces and a vehicle for navigating and reconstructing them. In particular, these cases explore the processes by which some bodies are stigmatized and others gain access to upward mobility and social benefit while also offering significant insights regarding how individuals experience and navigate their local body contexts—and, in turn, how those contexts affect their choices and outcomes.

THE MEANINGS OF FAT

A key concept engaged across the chapters is that of the "fat body" itself. What does it mean to be fat? Hruschka describes population-level obesity trends hinging on body mass index (BMI). Although BMI is a reasonable population measure, it falls short in accounting for differences in basal body mass across populations, sex differences, and individual differences. Commonly noted in the last category are variations in muscularity (e.g., where a person with above average muscle mass will appear as overweight or obese although they do not meet the health risk profile of someone whose mass is due to adiposity) and fat distribution (e.g., central adiposity, colloquially referred to as "apple shaped," will put someone at greater cardiovascular risk than hip distribution or "pear shaped"). These distinctions sometimes are reflected in socially desirable body ideals; examples include Taylor's US high school boys' aspirations for six-pack abs and Anderson-Fye et al.'s Jamaican college students' desire for hourglass-shaped women. In other words, social value judgments about fat hinge not only on *how much* fat a body has but also on *what kind* of fat, and in which configurations it appears. Social context, life stage, and everyday life roles also help shape the moral implications of fat.

Understanding the valuation of fat matters. If a person is the "wrong kind of fat," he or she may face substantial social penalty—for example, reduced opportunities for employment and marriage (Puhl and Heuer 2009). When this stigma is internalized, mental illnesses, including depression and eating disorders, become far more common (Friedman et al. 2005; Jackson, Grilo and Masheb 2000). Casper's and McClure's chapters unpack how intersectional positionalities—such as race and class—can further stigmatize individuals deemed to have undesirably fat bodies in the United States. In Casper's chapter, overweight pregnant women who are African American are singularly policed and blamed for high rates of infant mortality. The emphasis on monitoring obesity among African American pregnant women removes the focus from the more grave problem of high and disparate rates of infant mortality among African American women—rates that remain grossly unequal even when controlling for a myriad of variables including weight. McClure explains how racism persists in the "othering" of African American women in body image-related research. She turns W. E. B. Du Bois's powerful question—"How does it feel to be a problem?"—into an empirical one with African American young girls as they navigate body image in a US multiracial high school context. Rather than begin with etic categories derived from white girls, McClure uses the girls' experiences and categories to explain their physicality and embodied experiences. Their responses then offer opportunities for social critique. Each of these cases speaks to the social, psychological, and material consequences of fat stigma for those deemed to be or have the "wrong kind of fat."

Conversely, the right amount and/or kind of fat can lead to upward social mobility. Determining what is the optimal quantity and quality of fat in any given situation is complex but patterned (see also Anderson-Fye, McClure, and Wilson 2015). As a key instance, gender plays an important role in each of the contexts considered in these chapters, albeit in different ways. In Anderson-Fye et al.'s comparative research, for example, men were held to more exacting body standards than women in terms of heterosexual mate selection in Jamaica. In Belize, however, extra weight on males can appeal to potential mates, as a "good" chubby boyfriend was viewed as more likely to be a kind, caring, and faithful companion.

What counts as "good" or "bad" fat is not stable, however, and such valuations fluctuate. Although it is undeniably challenging to assess and explain the dynamics of the social valuation of fat and body ideals in a single limited context at one point in time, it is even more challenging to investigate trends under contexts of change. Nevertheless, several of these chapters expand and deepen our understanding of the roles globalization and transnational media play in this process around the world. Becker's work in Fiji and Trainer's in the UAE explain complex cases where, in the context of relatively large body sizes for women nationally, young women simultaneously grapple with global and local standards for body ideals and gendered comportment. Both examples demonstrate that global and local are no longer distinct. Constantly changing body standards for young women have crystallized moments where transnational or traditional standards come to the fore; nevertheless, these young women always navigate multiple markets and desired behaviors. Becker's participants solve the seemingly impossible conundrum of eating heartily like a "good Fijian" and maintaining a slender body akin to a Hollywood heroine by taking traditional herbal purgatives. They can behave like Fijians yet look like modern cosmopolitan women. And in the United Arab Emirates, young women attending university worry about weight with regard to their ability to attract romantic interest—and, in light of extensive gender segregation, are even more concerned with their peers' assessment of their appearance as they too grapple with being both traditional and modern.

These examples and others point toward innovation and agency within competing and constrained norms. How then, are we to understand theoretically the dynamics of body size, shape, and value that give rise to findings as diverse as those reported here? The cases described in this volume—from population-level to school-level micro-analysis—all engage what Edmonds and Mears call "body capital." In what follows, we reengage this concept in light of the empirical chapters to highlight both the benefits and limitations of adopting an economic model for understanding the social lives of bodies.

BODY CAPITAL REVISITED

As described above, body capital explains how different bodies carry different kinds of social value within local cultural, material, and moral worlds at particular points in time. The metaphor of capital is useful because it provides a language for discussing how bodies become signifiers of worth within broader networks. Specifically, it evokes the concept of a "market" through which the value of such capital is determined (see Edmonds and Mears in this volume for detailed discussion). However, the concept of "capital" also brings to the fore some of the challenges of using a market-based framework. By focusing on the constitution of different "body markets" and how the process of valuation happens, the chapters in this volume highlight the benefits and limitations of an economic paradigm for understanding body-image ideals and their implications. In doing so, they raise three provocative common themes: (1) issues of changing, hybrid, or multiple markets; (2) questions of moral dimensions of the body ideal beyond the Protestant ethic; and (3) the limits of an economic model for understanding body-image ideals. Each of these themes links questions of body capital to other social and cultural systems of value and worth.

Changing, Hybrid, and Multiple Markets

Several of the chapters emphasize that questions of body capital must be understood in the context of changing or multiple markets within which such capital is afforded value. For example, Edmonds and Mears argue that body capital is not determined simply by an abstract value of thinness as attractive and fatness as undesirable. Rather, social and cultural *processes* that are entangled with issues of labor, sexuality, leisure, and health combine to determine what kinds of bodies are considered attractive. In other words, Edmonds and Mears argue that what is valued are certain interpersonal and social *activities* that have as a natural byproduct a certain physiological outcome—rather than the corporeal aesthetic being the behavioral goal per se. This processual approach raises important questions when considering the values of thinness and fatness in a given context.

Although earlier authors have stressed that moral "goodness" tends to be associated with thinness and moral compromise with fatness (e.g., Bordo 1993), this relationship has generally remained framed within a discourse on beauty that considers the aesthetic dimension primary. Edmonds and Mears suggest that the aesthetic components of thinness or fatness (or the notions of thinness and fatness) as indicative of a person's individual moral composition may be secondary to what body size and shape are thought to signify about the individual's investment in the broader social community. This insight is revealed in examples such as Anderson-Fye et al.'s unexpected finding that some young Belizean women prefer a man with a potbelly as a future husband, even though belly rolls themselves were not considered attractive. Such women felt the presence of a potbelly evidenced a man's "good" moral activities and qualities, such as working hard and being humble, rather than a focus on exercise, presumably to stay attractive to other women. The more influential "market" for the thin body ideal, then, may be one predicated on prosociality rather than individual moral rectitude or physical attractiveness.

Similarly, Becker's work on rapid economic and social change in Fiji highlights the multiple "markets" within which girls' bodies are valued. Young women in particular become caught between the traditional valuing of eating, social obligations, and a larger body type and an upwardly mobile thinner shape. Being a good daughter and member of the community means eating heartily. To do otherwise reflects poorly not only on the girl but also on her family. At the same time, having an overweight body and not aspiring to a thinner ideal reflects poorly on a girl and carries negative real material implications for her family. Rather than simply pursuing a lean and toned body to demonstrate moral or social goodness, then, girls must navigate between opposing market values. In such a context, girls show their moral selves by eating well *and* keeping a svelte shape. These efforts affirm the logic of the marketplace by simultaneously working to stimulate the appetite and to rid the body of "excess" food or fat. What this means in everyday practice is that girls often feel challenged in a double bind and unable to satisfactorily meet the requirements of either measure of value.

Extending the theme of multiple markets and multiple forms of capital, Anderson-Fye et al.'s research emphasizes that a "thin" body ideal and a stigma against fat do not translate into identical preferences across countries or cultures. Both the *kind* of thin and the *kind* of fat matter in assessments of what bodies are considered acceptable or unacceptable. Even more, they argue, body-image concerns go beyond size and shape to encompass practices such as skin bleaching. Further, within different capitalist contexts, the rewards of attaining a local body ideal vary by setting—for example, depending on dance hall culture or the tourism industry. In short, not only does the value of the "thin body" differ, but so too do the kinds of thinness deemed ideal or the kind of fatness deemed problematic. In addition, thinness and fatness are not the only bodily aesthetics that affect value.

Taylor's chapter further highlights varying dimensions of aesthetic value by examining the different standards for boys and girls regarding thinness and fatness, how such markets are linguistically and discursively generated and monitored, and with what implications. Although both boys and girls feel pressure to adhere to local standards of ideal body types, she notes, the practical implications of that pressure vary. Boys, for example, can wear baggy clothes, whereas girls are expected to wear clothes that leave them "nowhere to hide." And although boys may gain capital by having six packs, they retain the choice over whether to offer them for display. In other words, simply considering the presence or absence of a certain body ideal does not capture the full range of social and cultural practices that bear on the attainment and demonstration of that ideal.

In considering the body as capital, then, these chapters highlight the complexities of the marketplaces within which the body is valued. Specifically, they consider how marketplaces change or fluctuate depending on the context, revealing local tensions, concerns, and contradictions that are worked out through the ways in which bodies are valued and capitalized in the social arena, as well as how individuals navigate multilevel dynamics.

MORAL DIMENSIONS BEYOND THE PROTESTANT ETHIC

Despite different geographic and topical focuses, each of these chapters engages the prevailing assumption that a thin body ideal and a stigma against fat is a unique feature of late capitalist development. Theorists such as Susan Bordo (1993) have posited that this association stems from capitalism's Protestant ethic and the moral value of self-denial to achieve future aims. Although this understanding is still prevalent in arguments about capitalism and body image (and appears in some of the chapters here), cross-cultural work such as that featured in this collection shows that the situation on the ground is significantly more complex.

One of the problems with earlier theorizing on the thin body ideal's relationship to capitalism is the assumption that the thin body's worth is the same—and carries the same meaning—everywhere. In other words, the "capitalism-equals-thin-ideal-and-fat-stigma" argument assumes a homogeneity of capitalist systems and perspectives on thinness and fatness that empirical research does not support. In fact, as just discussed, the value of the "thin body ideal" fluctuates and gains different degrees of purchase in different places at different times, depending on other aspects of the local body economy. Positing an understanding of the link between capitalism and a preference for thinness as necessarily indicating a shared moral project is therefore highly problematic.

This variation in the meanings of thinness and fatness does not, however, mean that no shared moral projects exist, simply that they are not reducible to the "thin = good" and "fat = bad" propositions as naturalized assumptions. In addressing this issue, these chapters demonstrate that modes of participation may serve as domains of negotiating moral self-making. That is, people participate *both* in capital (as bodies to be valued) *and* in markets (as subjects who do the valuing). These dual processes engage strategies for being seen as a good person by others and by oneself. People living in and with bodies do not experience those bodies simply as capital alone; in living their own conditions of embodiment, each person becomes part of the "marketplace" for others, albeit with differential power. It is this "both/and" dynamic that is perhaps more characteristic of capitalist economic systems than a codified preference for thinness per se.

Taylor's work, for example, shows how moral participation is demonstrated not only in meeting an ideal but also in measuring *others* against this ideal in social interactions. The latter involves moral positioning through evaluative commentary on others, communicating not only with words but also through tone. McClure's chapter shows how African American women's experiences of body image are rendered exceptional and marginalized when they engage multiple "marketplace" standards not well represented in dominant discourse or scientific frames. Her empirical work aims to articulate multifaceted body projects of African American high school girls that, rather than "exceptions" to white girls' categories, hold great internally consistent moral logic.

Anderson-Fye et al. come at this question from another perspective, looking not so much at how thinness is valued but how fat is stigmatized. Their research found that fat stigma is present even in supposedly fat-loving cultures. As in Taylor's chapter, the ways in which people position themselves as arbiters of *other* people's worth based on body size become an important means of constituting themselves as certain kinds of moral actors.

In Trainer's study, meanwhile, young women in university in the UAE see longstanding demographic trends of great wealth and prevalence of overweight and obesity among women over thirty. At the same time, however, they experience and express common peer perspectives regarding the importance of thin bodies to attracting romantic interest and maintaining approval among their classmates. In earlier generations, plumpness prompted positive reactions, yet these women now found their parents encouraging self-discipline—thin daughters reflected well upon them as caregivers. Not unlike the young women in Becker's Fijian study, they must operate in simultaneously disjunctive and ambivalent contexts to craft their own and others' moral positionality.

Hruschka's chapter highlights this overdetermination of the relationship between capital and markets by highlighting various interpretations that can be brought to bear on the correlation between high socioeconomic status (SES) and lower BMI. He explores questions of whether more resources translate to more opportunities to attain thinness, whether thinness allows a person to obtain more resources, and what, if anything, these links would tell us about the relationship between economic development and body-ideal preferences.

How we understand the association between SES and thinness is critically important, as it goes to the heart of the causal link assumed between capitalism and the thin body ideal. Over time, the body that takes greater resources has been considered desirable (Anderson-Fye 2012). It has generally been accepted in the literature (Hesse-Biber 1996; Gerber and Quinn 2008; Mendelson et al. 2002) that thinness is valued in capitalist systems and being thin allows one to "barter" one's body capital for access to greater resources. This presumption is part of why thinness has been perceived as an "aspirational" state, a means to achieve a higher standard of living, and fat has been stigmatized. But with greater access to resources and more leisure time, individuals are better able to obtain and maintain the body that is most valued in a given context. How, then, can we posit a causative argument?

The challenge of this sort of macro-engagement is that it risks linking body capital (thinness) to economic resources in a way that implicitly assumes that thinness is the item of value rather than other practices (such as exercise or moderation in consumption) that are correlated with thinness. Thus Edmonds and Mears argue what is considered attractive may have less to do with the specifics of the body and more to do with the local meanings of the practices that result in thinness. This theoretical shift leads to additional questions. For example, why do we assume that female thinness is the dependent variable? What if male wealth and female thinness co-create? Here we might recall Becker's piece about how the female body is not just a resource of the individual but of families. How do women's bodies become community property within heterosexual relationships? How is this paralleled with men's earning potential? For example, does having a thinner female partner signal something to other men (and women) about a man's business acumen or promise for success? Might the body capital of the female partner in a relationship "rub off" on the male as supposed evidence of his capacity for achievement? If so, might this translate into greater opportunities for him to advance socially and financially? In this regard, it might be the case that the cultivation of an ideal body type by a female partner enables or enhances a male partner's economic success in a way that is not captured by the traditional understandings of thinness as something to be bartered directly for material resources.

McClure's rendering of the long history of othering African American women's bodies would also seem to support a shift to focus on practice not product of beauty ideals. McClure explains that the research literature has found that African American women have less body dissatisfaction than women in other racial groups yet also have high rates of obesity. In a singular body product–based theory of symbolic body capital where, to the extent that one matches the slender cultural ideals, one gains upward mobility, the situation among African American women is unintelligible. Instead, McClure points out that both positive body image and weight concern coexist among African American women. From an emic point of view, this coexistence is reconcilable through contingent and intersectional experiences of individual women in their historical, political, social, and economic contexts.

Taken together, these chapters productively challenge the prevailing view that thinness is an avenue for the attainment and expression of moral personhood within capitalist systems and fatness is necessarily stigmatized in predictable ways. In this model, thinness represents adherence to the values of delayed gratification and therefore signals a moral rectitude that is prized as the purview of the elect, whereas fatness signals an unwillingness or inability to live up to such moral ideals. The chapters here suggest an expanded perspective, in that how people position themselves as members of the marketplace can have just as much moral valence as how they position themselves as "capital" within such structures of value. How people evaluate others' bodies says just as much about them as moral persons as how their own bodies are evaluated by others.

Limitations of the Economic Model

In addition to extending and elaborating upon existing understandings of the links between capitalism, the thin body ideal, and fat stigma, these chapters further highlight several limitations of the economic model for thinking about body image. Using an economic paradigm as an analytic framework for accounting for aesthetic preferences, for example, subsumes discussions of thinness and fatness into the logic space of capitalism before an analysis has taken place. As a result, it becomes difficult to imagine conclusions that counter capitalist assumptions. In this regard, Becker's work in Fiji offers evidence and insights that inform a reassessment of those assumptions.

In her chapter, Becker argues that body agency is not the property of the individual but the responsibility of the family. This perspective can lead to excessive monitoring of children's eating and growth because the "good family" produces a body that reflects good care. In Fiji, good care is shown by a heavier body type, even though it is not rated most attractive. Becker's analysis suggests that a strict application of a capitalist model to understandings of body ideals is inadequate for the complexity of factors and processes that form those ideals. In fact, Becker demonstrates, multiple and even conflicting measures of value can be operating simultaneously. In addition, she notes that people do not necessarily function as "free agents" within these markets in the ways that capitalist economic theories presume.

Much of Becker's explanation about Fiji can be applied productively to children in the United States, albeit with different cultural meanings. From the moment their children are born, American parents hear that they must monitor and regulate their child's appetite and eating. The prevalence of such messages increase as children get older, including exhortations to offer only organic foods, ensure they eat their vegetables, or enroll them in athletic programs. Given this context, parents understandably can feel that they have an active stake in the attractiveness of children's bodies — and in fact, that their children's bodies are evidence of the competence of their parenting.

In the realm of eating disorders, such involvement can be pathologized and called *enmeshment*. Parental over-investment in their child's appearance is often seen as a contributor to the development of eating disorders in the first place. At the same time, children's insistence that *they* are the bosses of their own bodies is targeted as an obsession with control that must be alleviated in the course of treatment. This ambivalent body agency is visible in family-based treatments for anorexia nervosa, where parents take responsibility for refeeding the child.

In addition to ambivalent body agency, the capitalist model is challenged when the markets (here, employment and marriage) do not work as they are supposed to do. For example, in Anderson-Fye et al.'s research in Nepal, although ample evidence suggested that slender bodies did better in employment markets, the data were inconsistent for marriage markets. In fact, the data showed that young people were confused about what—if anything—body type had to do with mate selection. College students could not answer survey questions when shown a body figures scale and asked which body type would make the best spouse. Of over one hundred respondents, the vast majority called over the researchers to attempt to explain the question or left it blank. These young people from many backgrounds in Nepal could easily pick out which body shape would succeed in a workplace. But they saw no association between body size and the character and social traits that would make someone a good or desirable spouse. In this instance, of the two dominant markets described in Hruschka's chapter (i.e., employment and marriage), one of them lacked the validity to be considered.

In short, competing understandings of body agency and moral value exist around the world. Naturalizing as "Western" a body capital framework that posits clear markets and rational actors—and against which other frameworks are compared—sets up an empirically false premise that colors not only the interpretation of data but also our very strategies and priorities of investigation.

These chapters have shown that markets are complex and variable, with different capital value associated with different body types and body behaviors in different circumstances. If management of the body is never strictly an individualist enterprise but always involves shared moral implications, then body ideals emerge from more than individual rational actor assumptions that underlie economic theory.

CONCLUSION

Taken together, the chapters in this volume demonstrate both the utility and challenges of our inherited epistemological frameworks for thinking about culture and body image. In doing so, they productively push on received assumptions and categories, signaling alternate directions for investigation and new avenues for growth. Notably, they remind us that "one size does not fit all" in theoretical explication of global obesity and body-image trends any more than it does in body ideals. At the same time, crosscutting patterns and driving processes are important to consider. As Brewis highlights in the introduction, this volume includes multilevel analyses. Working across levels is crucial to understanding both widespread patterns and key variations, a classical goal of anthropological study.

In particular, this volume reminds us of the dynamism of our analytic concepts. Terms such as *body, capital, market, fat,* and *thin* are too frequently treated as static signifiers in this realm of work. The chapters here provide vivid evidence of the importance of positionality and contextual analysis for each. More, the processes and practices by which some bodies are valued and some are stigmatized are highlighted as at least as important as the end products.

The implications of expanding our analytic tools and subsequent understandings are paramount on a fat planet. Unquestionably, "globesity" is an issue increasingly compromising health in populations around the world. However, in our urge to seize obesity as a public health problem, we already have evidence of iatrogenic effect (e.g., Brewis 2015; Greenhalgh 2015). It is our hope that through nuanced investigations and considerations, such as those in this volume, more careful and accurate interventions can be designed for health promotion. Far from the antiquated conceptualization of "cultural competence" in which cultures were considered discrete entities and treatments oversimplified, the chapters here point to both important global trends (such as shared media images or tourism) and key specificities (such as religious beliefs or particular histories of racism) that matter on the ground in people's everyday lives. With as multifaceted and complex an issue as weight-related attitudes are known to be, our investigations must remain diligent and in conversation across levels and locations as endeavored here.

ABRAMS, KAY KOSAK, LA RUE ALLEN, AND JAMES GRAY

1993   "Disordered Eating Attitudes and Behaviors, Psychological Adjustment, and Ethnic Identity: A Comparison of Black and White Female College Students." *International Journal of Eating Disorders* 14 (1): 49–57.

ABU-LUGHOD, LILA

1993   *Writing Women's Worlds: Bedouin Stories.* Berkeley and Los Angeles: University of California Press.

AKAN, GLORIA E., AND CARLOS M. GRILO

1995   "Sociocultural Influences on Eating Attitudes and Behaviors, Body-Image, and Psychological Functioning: A Comparison of African-American, Asian-American, and Caucasian College-Women." *International Journal of Eating Disorders* 18 (2): 181–87.

ALEXANDER, MICHELLE

2010   *The New Jim Crow: Mass Incarceration in the Age of Colorblindness.* New York: New Press.

AL JAZEERA

2013   "America's Infant Mortality Crisis." *AlJazeera.com*, September 26. http://www.aljazeera.com/programmes/faultlines/2013/09/20139248355279581.html.

ALLAN, JANET D., KELLY MAYO, AND YVONNE MICHEL

1993   "Body Size Values of White and Black Women." *Research in Nursing & Health* 16 (5): 323–33.

ALMEIDA, LILIANA, SARAH SAVOY, AND PAUL BOXER

2011   "The Role of Weight Stigmatization in Cumulative Risk for Binge Eating." *Journal of Clinical Psychology* 67 (3): 278–92.

AL-QASIMI, NOOR

2010   "Immodest Modesty: Accommodating Dissent and the 'Abaya-as-Fashion' in the Arab Gulf States." *Journal of Middle East Women's Studies* 6 (1): 46–74.

AL-SHAREKH, ALANOUD, ED.

2007   *The Gulf Family: Kinship Policies and Modernity.* London: SAQI Books and the London Middle East Institute.

AL-SHAREKH, ALANOUD, AND ROBERT SPRINGBORG, EDS.

2008   *Popular Culture and Political Identity in the Arab Gulf States.* London: SAQI Books and the London Middle East Institute.

AMERICAN PSYCHIATRIC ASSOCIATION (APA)

2000   *Diagnostic and Statistical Manual of Mental Disorders.* 4th ed. Arlington, VA: American Psychiatric Association.

ANDERSON, BENEDICT

1983   *Imagined Communities: Reflections on the Origin and Spread of Nationalism.* London: Verso.

ANDERSON, TAMMY L., CATHERINE GRUNERT, ARIELLE KATZ, AND
SAMANTHA LOVASCIO

2010   "Aesthetic Capital: A Research Review on Beauty Perks and Penalties." *Sociology Compass* 4 (8): 564–75.

ANDERSON-FYE, EILEEN

2004   "A Coca-Cola Shape: Cultural Change, Body Image, and Eating Disorders in San Andrés, Belize." *Culture, Medicine, and Psychiatry* 28 (4): 561–95.

2011   "Body Images in Non-Western Cultures." In *Body Image: A Handbook of Science, Practice, and Prevention*, edited by Thomas F. Cash and Linda Smolak. New York: Guilford.

2012   "Anthropological Perspectives on Physical Appearance and Body Image." In *Encyclopedia of Body Image and Human Appearance*, edited by Thomas F. Cash, 15–22. New York: Academic Press.

ANDERSON-FYE, EILEEN P., AND ARUNDATI BHARATI

n.d.   *In and Out of the Robe: Piety and Embodiment in a Nepali Monastery.* Global Fat Stigma Working Paper.

ANDERSON-FYE, EILEEN P., AND JERRY FLOERSCH

2011   "I'm Not Your Typical 'Homework Stresses Me Out' Kind of Girl: Psychological Anthropology in Research on College Students' Usage of Psychiatric Medications and Mental Health Services." *Ethos* 39 (4): 501–21.

ANDERSON-FYE, EILEEN P., AND JIELU LIN

2009   "Belief and Behavior Aspects of the EAT-26: The Case of Schoolgirls in Belize." *Culture, Medicine, and Psychiatry* 33 (4): 623–38.

ANDERSON-FYE, EILEEN, STEPHANIE MCCLURE, AND RACHEL WILSON

2015   "Cultural Similarities and Differences in Eating Disorders." In *Handbook of Eating Disorders*, edited by Linda Smolak and Michael Levine, 297–311. Hoboken, NJ: Wiley-Blackwell.

ANDREYEVA, TATIANA, REBECCA M. PUHL, AND KELLY D. BROWNELL

2008   "Changes in Perceived Weight Discrimination among Americans, 1995–1996 through 2004–2006." *Obesity* 16 (5): 1129–34.

ANTIN, TAMAR M. J., AND GEOFFREY HUNT

2013   "Embodying both Stigma and Satisfaction: An Interview Study of African American Women." *Critical Public Health* 23 (1): 17–31.

ARMSTRONG, DAVID
1986   "The Invention of Infant Mortality." *Sociology of Health and Illness* 8:211–32.

ATRASH, HANI K., KAY JOHNSON, MYRON (MIKE) ADAMS, JOSÉ F. CORDERO, AND
JENNIFER HOWSE
2006   "Preconception Care for Improving Perinatal Outcomes: The Time to Act."
         Maternal and Child Health Journal 10:S3–S11.

AVERETT, SUSAN L., AND SANDERS KORENMAN
1996   "The Economic Reality of the Beauty Myth." *Journal of Human Resources*
         31 (2): 304–30.

AVERETT, SUSAN L., ASIA SIKORA, AND LAURA M. ARGYS
2008   "For Better or Worse: Relationship Status and Body Mass Index. *Economics
         & Human Biology* 6 (3): 330–49.

AVERETT, SUSAN L., AND JULIE K. SMITH
2013   "Financial Hardship and Obesity." *Economics & Human Biology*.

BARKER, D. J. P.
1997   "Maternal Nutrition, Fetal Nutrition, and Disease in Later Life." *Nutrition*
         13:807.

BARKER, KRISTIN K.
1998   "A Ship upon a Stormy Sea: The Medicalization of Pregnancy." *Social Science
         and Medicine* 47 (8): 1067–76.

BARRY, COLLEEN L., VICTORIA L. BRESCOLL, KELLY D. BROWNELL, AND
MARK SCHLESINGER
2009   "Obesity Metaphors: How Beliefs about the Causes of Obesity Affect Support
         for Public Policy." *Milbank Quarterly* 87 (1): 7–47.

BARTKY, SANDRA
1990   *Femininity and Domination.* New York: Routledge.

BASHFORD, ALISON, AND CLAIRE HOOKER, EDS.
2001   *Contagion: Historical and Cultural Studies.* London: Routledge.

BASS, MARGARET K.
2001   "On Being a Fat Black Girl in a Fat-Hating Culture." In *Recovering the Black
         Female Body: Self-Representations by African American Women,* edited by
         Michael Bennett and Vanessa D. Dickerson, 219–30. New Brunswick, NJ:
         Rutgers University Press.

BATURKA, NATALIE, PAIGE P. HORNSBY, AND JOHN B. SCHORLING
2000   "Clinical Implications of Body Image among Rural African American
         Women." *Journal of General Internal Medicine* 15 (4): 235–41.

BECKER, ANNE E.
1994   "Nurturing and Negligence: Working on Others' Bodies in Fiji." In

Embodiment and Experience: The Existential Ground of Culture and Self, edited by Thomas J. Csordas, 100–115. Cambridge: Cambridge University Press.

1995   *Body, Self, and Society: The View from Fiji*. Philadelphia: University of Pennsylvania Press.

1997   "Pregnant Bodies and Interpersonal Boundaries in Fiji." *Domodomo: Fiji Museum Quarterly* 11:25–32.

1998   "Postpartum Illness in Fiji: A Sociosomatic Perspective." *Psychosomatic Medicine* 60 (4): 431–38.

2003   "Eating Disorders and Social Transition." *Primary Psychiatry* 10:75–79.

2004   "Television, Disordered Eating, and Young Women in Fiji: Negotiating Body Image and Identity during Rapid Social Change." *Culture, Medicine, and Psychiatry* 28:533–59.

2013   "Resocializing Body Weight, Obesity, and Health Agency." In *The Meaning of Measures, the Measures of Meaning: Reconstructing Obesity Research*, edited by Megan McCullough and Jessica Hardin, 27–48. New York: Berghahn Books.

BECKER, ANNE E., ASENACA BAINIVUALIKU, A. NISHA KHAN, W. AALBERSBERG, P. GERAGHTY, STEPHEN E. GILMAN, ANDREA L. ROBERTS, KESAIA NAVARA, LAUREN K. RICHARDS, ALEXANDRA PERLOE, E. V. BERESIN, AND RUTH H. STRIEGEL-MOORE
2009   "Feasibility of a School-based Study of Health Risk Behaviors in Ethnic Fijian Female Adolescents in Fiji: The HEALTHY Fiji Study." *Fiji Medical Journal* 28:18–34.

BECKER, ANNE E., REBECCA A. BURWELL, STEPHEN E. GILMAN, DAVID B. HERZOG, AND PAUL HAMBURG
2002   "Eating Behaviors and Attitudes Following Prolonged Television Exposure among Ethnic Fijian Adolescent Girls." *British Journal of Psychiatry* 180: 509–14.

BECKER, ANNE E., KRISTEN FAY, JESSICA AGNEW-BLAIS, PETER M. GUARNACCIA, RUTH H. STRIEGEL-MOORE, AND STEPHEN E. GILMAN
2010a   "Development of a Measure of 'Acculturation' for Ethnic Fijians: Methodologic and Conceptual Considerations for Application to Eating Disorders Research." *Transcultural Psychiatry* 47 (5): 754–88.

BECKER, ANNE E., KRISTEN FAY, JESSICA AGNEW-BLAIS, A. NISHA KHAN, RUTH H. STRIEGEL-MOORE, AND STEPHEN E. GILMAN
2011   "Social Network Media Exposure and Adolescent Eating Pathology in Fiji." *British Journal of Psychiatry* 2011 198 (1): 43–50.

BECKER, ANNE E., STEPHEN E. GILMAN, AND REBECCA A. BURWELL

2005   "Changes in Prevalence of Overweight and in Body Image among Fijian
        Women between 1989 and 1998." *Obesity Research* 13 (1): 110–17.

BECKER, ANNE E., AND JENNIFER J. THOMAS

2015   "Eating Pathology in Fiji: Phenomenologic Diversity, Visibility, and Vulnera-
        bility." In *Revisioning Psychiatry: Cultural Phenomenology, Critical Neuro-
        science, and Global Mental Health,* edited by Laurence J. Kirmayer, Robert
        Lemelson, and Constance A. Cummings, 515–43. Cambridge: Cambridge
        University Press.

BECKER, ANNE E., JENNIFER J. THOMAS, ASENACA BAINIVUALIKU, LAUREN RICHARDS,
KESAIA NAVARA, ANDREA L. ROBERTS, STEPHEN E. GILMAN, AND
RUTH H. STRIEGEL-MOORE

2010b   "Adaptation and Evaluation of the Clinical Impairment Assessment to Assess
        Disordered Eating Related Distress in an Adolescent Female Ethnic Fijian
        Population." *International Journal of Eating Disorders* 43:179–86.

BEN-TOVIM, DAVID I.

1996   "Is Big Still Beautiful in Polynesia?" *Lancet* 348:1047–48.

BERLANT, LAUREN

2007   "Slow Death (Sovereignty, Obesity, Lateral Agency)." *Critical Inquiry* 33 (4):
        754–80.

BERNARD, H. RUSSELL, AND CLARENCE GRAVLEE, EDS.

2014   *Handbook of Methods in Cultural Anthropology.* 2nd ed. Latham, MD: Row-
        man and Littlefield.

BERNSTEIN, ELIZABETH

2007   *Temporarily Yours: Intimacy, Authenticity, and the Commerce of Sex.* Chicago:
        University of Chicago Press.

BHARATI, ARUNDHATI, AND EILEEN ANDERSON-FYE

n.d.   *Mind and Body in Modern Contemplative Life: Body Ideals among a Group of
        Nepali Buddhist Monks.* Global Fat Stigma Working Paper.

BILTEKOFF, CHARLOTTE

2007   "The Terror Within: Obesity in Post 9/11 U.S. Life." *American Studies* 48 (3):
        29–48.

BINDON, JAMES R., AND PAUL T. BAKER

1985   "Modernization, Migration and Obesity among Samoan Adults." *Annals of
        Human Biology* 12:67–76.

BISSELL, KIMBERLY L.

2002   "I Want to Be Thin, Like You." *Visual Communication Quarterly* 9 (2): 4–11.

BLACK, MAUREEN M., MIA A. PAPAS, MARGARET E. BENTLEY, PAMELA CURETON,
ALICIA SAUNDERS, KATHERINE LE, JEAN ANLIKER, AND NONI ROBINSON

2006   "Overweight Adolescent African-American Mothers Gain Weight in Spite of
        Intentions to Lose Weight." *Journal of the American Dietetic Association* 106
        (1): 80–87.

BLEICH, S. N., R. J. THORPE, H. SHARIF-HARRIS, F. FESAHAZION, AND T. A. LAVEIST

2010   "Social Context Explains Race Disparities in Obesity Among Women." *Jour-
        nal of Epidemiology and Community Health* 64 (5): 465–69.

BOERO, NATALIE

2007   "All the News That's Fat to Print: The American 'Obesity Epidemic' and the
        Media." *Qualitative Sociology* 30 (1): 41–60.

2010   "Bypassing Blame: Bariatric Surgery and the Case of Biomedical Failure."
        In *Biomedicalization: Technoscience, Health, and Illness in the U.S.*, edited by
        Adele E. Clarke, Laura Mamo, Jennifer Ruth Fosket, Jennifer R. Fishman,
        and Janet K. Shim, 307–30. Durham, NC: Duke University Press.

2012   *Killer Fat: Media, Medicine, and Morals in the American "Obesity Epidemic."*
        New Brunswick, NJ: Rutgers University Press.

BORDO, SUSAN

1993   *Unbearable Weight: Feminism, Western Culture, and the Body.* Berkeley and
        Los Angeles: University of California Press.

1999   *The Male Body: A New Look at Men in Public and in Private.* New York:
        Farrar, Straus and Giroux.

BOTTA, RENEE A.

2000   "The Mirror of Television: A Comparison of Black and White Adolescents'
        Body Image." *Journal of Communication* 50 (3): 144–59.

BOURDIEU, PIERRE

1977 [1972]   *Outline of a Theory of Practice.* Translated by Richard Nice. Cambridge:
        Cambridge University Press.

1984   *Distinction: A Social Critique of the Judgment of Taste.* Cambridge: Harvard
        University Press.

1986   "The Forms of Capital." In *Handbook of Theory and Research for the Soci-
        ology of Education*, edited by J. G. Richardson, 241–58. New York: Green-
        wood Press.

1990   *The Logic of Practice.* Translated by Richard Nice. Stanford, CA: Stanford
        University Press.

1993   *The Field of Cultural Production: Essays on Art and Literature.* New York:
        Columbia University Press.

BOZOYAN, CHRISTIANE, AND TOBIAS WOLBRING
2011   "Fat, Muscles, and Wages." *Economics & Human Biology* 9 (4): 356–63.

BREWIS, ALEXANDRA A.
2011   *Obesity: Cultural and Biocultural Perspectives.* New Brunswick, NJ: Rutgers University Press.
2014   "Stigma and the Perpetuation of Obesity." *Social Science and Medicine* 118: 152–58.

BREWIS, ALEXANDRA A., DANIEL J. HRUSCHKA, AND AMBER WUTICH
2011   "Vulnerability to Fat-Stigma in Women's Everyday Relationships." *Social Science and Medicine* 73:491–97.

BREWIS, ALEXANDRA A., AND STEPHEN T. MCGARVEY
2000   "Body Image, Body Size, and Samoan Ecological and Individual Moderniza-tion." *Ecology of Food and Nutrition* 39:105–20.

BREWIS, ALEXANDRA A., STEPHEN T. MCGARVEY, J. JONES, AND BOYD A. SWINBURN
1998   "Perceptions of Body Size in Pacific Islanders." *International Journal of Obesity* 22 (2): 185–89.

BREWIS, ALEXANDRA A., AND AMBER WUTICH
2011   "Vulnerability to Fat-Stigma in Women's Everyday Relationships." *Social Science and Medicine* 73:491–97.
2012   "Implicit versus Explicit Fat-Stigma." *American Journal of Human Biology* 24:332–38.
2014   "A World of Suffering? Biocultural Approaches to Fat Stigma in the Global Contexts of the Obesity Epidemic." *Annals of Anthropological Practice* 38 (2): 269–83.

BREWIS, ALEXANDRA A., AMBER WUTICH, ASHLAN FALETTA-COWDEN, AND
ISA RODRIGUEZ-SOTO
2011   "Body Norms and Fat Stigma in Global Perspective." *Current Anthropology* 52:269–76.

BRISTOL-RHYS, JANE
2010   *Emirati Women: Generations of Change.* New York: Columbia University Press.

BRITTON, LAUREN E., DENISE M. MARTZ, DORIS G. BAZZINI, LISA A. CURTIN, AND
ANNI LEASHOMB
2006   "Fat Talk and Self-Presentation of Body Image: Is There a Social Norm for Women to Self-Degrade?" *Body Image* 3 (3): 247–54.

BROOKE, R. C., S. J. SIMPSON, AND D. RAUBENHEIMER
2010   "The Price of Protein: Combining Evolutionary and Economic Analysis to Understanding Excessive Energy Consumption." *Obesity Reviews* 11 (12): 887–94.

BROWN, P. J., AND M. KONNER

1987   "An Anthropological Perspective on Obesity." *Annals of the New York Academy of Sciences* 499 (1): 29–46.

BROWNELL, KELLY D., AND KATHERINE BATTLE HORGEN

2004   *Food Fight: The Inside Story of the Food Industry, America's Obesity Crisis, and What We Can Do about It.* Chicago: Contemporary Books.

BROWNELL, KELLY D., ROGAN KERSH, DAVID S. LUDWIG, ROBERT C. POST, REBECCA M. PUHL, MARLENE B. SCHWARTZ, AND WALTER C. WILLETT

2010   "Personal Responsibility and Obesity: A Constructivist Approach to a Controversial Issue." *Health Affairs* 29 (3): 379–87.

BROWNELL, KELLY D., AND REBECCA M. PUHL

2003   "Stigma and Discrimination in Weight Management and Obesity." *Permanente Journal* 7 (3): 21–23.

BROWNELL, KELLY, REBECCA PUHL, MARLENE SCHWARTZ, AND LESLIE RUDD, EDS.

2005   *Weight Bias: Nature, Consequences, and Remedies.* New York: Guilford.

BROWNELL, SUSAN

2005   "China Reconstructs: Cosmetic Surgery and Nationalism in the Reform Era." In *Asian Medicine and Globalization*, edited by Joseph Alter. Philadelphia: University of Philadelphia Press.

BRUMBERG, JOAN JACOBS

1988   *Fasting Girls: The Emergence of Anorexia Nervosa as a Modern Disease.* Cambridge: Harvard University Press.

1989   *Fasting Girls: The History of Anorexia Nervosa.* New York: Plume.

1997   *The Body Project: An Intimate History of American Girls.* New York: Vintage Books.

BUCHOLTZ, MARY, AND KIRA HALL

2005   "Identity and Interaction: A Sociocultural Linguistic Approach." *Discourse Studies* 7 (4–5): 585–614.

BURNS, CATE

2004   *A Review of the Literature Describing the Link between Poverty, Food Insecurity and Obesity with Specific Reference to Australia.* Melbourne: Victorian Health Promotion Foundation.

BUTLER, JUDITH

1993   *Bodies that Matter: On the Discursive Limits of "Sex."* New York: Routledge.

CALIENDO, MARCO, AND WANG-SHENG LEE

2013   "Fat Chance! Obesity and the Transition from Unemployment to Employment." *Economics & Human Biology* 11 (2): 121–33.

CAMPBELL, NANCY D.

1999   "Regulating 'Maternal Instinct': Governing Mentalities of Late Twentieth-Century U.S. Illicit Drug Policy." *Signs* 24 (4): 895–923.

CAMPOS, PAUL, ABIGAIL SAGUY, PAUL ERNSBERGER, ERIC OLIVER, AND
GLENN GAESSER

2006   "The Epidemiology of Overweight and Obesity: Public Health Crisis or Moral Panic?" *International Journal of Epidemiology* 35 (1): 55–60.

CANGUILHEM, GEORGES

1991 [1978]   *The Normal and the Pathological*. Cambridge, MA: Zone Books.

CARPENTER, KENNETH M., DEBORAH S. HASIN, DAVID B. ALLISON, AND
MYLES S. FAITH

2000   "Relationships between Obesity and DSM-IV Major Depressive Disorder, Suicide Ideation, and Suicide Attempts: Results from a General Population Study." *American Journal of Public Health* 90:251–57.

CARPENTER, LAURA M., AND MONICA J. CASPER

2009   "Global Intimacies: Innovating the HPV Vaccine for Women's Health." *Women's Studies Quarterly* 37 (1/2): 80–100.

CARRYER, JENNIFER

1997   "A Feminist Appraisal of the Experience of Embodied Largeness: A Challenge for Nursing." PhD diss., Massey University.

CASPER, MONICA J.

1998a   *The Making of the Unborn Patient: A Social Anatomy of Fetal Surgery*. New Brunswick, NJ: Rutgers University Press.

1998b   "Working On and Around Human Fetuses: The Contested Domain of Fetal Surgery." In *Differences in Medicine: Unraveling Practices, Techniques, and Bodies*, edited by Marc Berg and Annemarie Mol, 28–52. Durham, NC: Duke University Press.

2010   "Phantom Babies and Spectral Women: Infant Mortality, Maternal/Child Health, and Women's Empowerment." Paper presented at a meeting of the American Anthropological Association, New Orleans, November 20.

2013a   "Biopolitics of Infant Mortality." *Anthropologies*, March 15. http://www.anthropologiesproject.org/2013/03/biopolitics-of-infant-mortality.html.

2013b   "The Infant Mortality Rate as Portable Abacus." Paper presented at the School of Sociology Brownbag Series, University of Arizona, March 8.

2014   "Abject(ified) Reproduction." *Hysteria* 3. http://hystericalfeminisms.com.

CASPER, MONICA J., AND LAURA M. CARPENTER

2008   "Sex, Drugs, and Politics: The HPV Vaccine for Cervical Cancer." *Sociology of Health and Illness* 30 (6): 886–99.

CASPER, MONICA J., AND LISA JEAN MOORE

2009   *Missing Bodies: The Politics of Visibility*. New York: New York University
        Press.

CASPER, MONICA J., AND LYNN M. MORGAN

2004   "Constructing Fetal Citizens." *Anthropology News* 45:17–18.

CASPER, MONICA J., AND WILLIAM PAUL SIMMONS

2014   "Accounting for Death: Infant Mortality, the MDGs, and Women's (Dis)
        Empowerment." In *Counting on Marilyn Waring: New Advances in Femi-
        nist Economics*, edited by Margunn Bjørnholt and Alisa McKay. Bradford,
        Ontario: Demeter Press.

CASPER, MONICA J., AND HEATHER LAINE TALLEY

2007   "Feminist Disability Studies." In *The Encyclopedia of Sociology*, edited by
        George Rizer. Hoboken, NJ: Wiley-Blackwell.

CASTELLS, MANUEL

1997   *The Information Age: Economy, Society and Culture*. Vol. 2 of *The Power of
        Identity*. Cambridge, MA: Blackwell.

CAWLEY, JOHN, JOHN MORAN, AND KOSALI SIMON

2010   "The Impact of Income on the Weight of Elderly Americans." *Health Eco-
        nomics* 19 (8): 979–93.

CENTERS FOR DISEASE CONTROL AND PREVENTION (CDC)

n.d.   "Body Mass Index (BMI)." Centers for Disease Control and Prevention,
        http:www.cdc.gov/healthyweight/assessing/BMI. Accessed May 2015.

2009   "Differences in Prevalence of Obesity among Black, White, and Hispanic
        Adults — United States, 2006–2008." *MMWR* 58 (27): 740–44.

CHANG, V. W., AND D. S. LAUDERDALE

2005   "Income Disparities in Body Mass Index and Obesity in the United States,
        1971–2002." *Archives of Internal Medicine* 165:2122–28.

CHARLES, DEBORAH

2012   "Pentagon Attacks Obesity with New Food Choices." Reuters, February 9.
        http://www.reuters.com/article/2012/02/09/us-usa-military-obesity
        -idUSTRE8180RV20120209. Accessed March 2, 2015.

CHAY, KENNETH Y., AND MICHAEL GREENSTONE

2000   "The Convergence in Black-White Infant Mortality during the 1960s."
        American Economic Review 90 (2): 326–32.

CHEN, AIMIN, SHINGAIRAI A. FERESU, CRISTINA FERNANDEZ, AND WALTER J. ROGAN

2009   "Maternal Obesity and the Risk of Infant Death in the United States." *Epi-
        demiology* 20:74–81.

CHIAPPORI, PIERRE-ANDRÉ, SONIA OREFFICE, AND CLIMENT QUINTANA-DOMEQUE

2012   "Fatter Attraction: Anthropometric and Socioeconomic Matching on the Marriage Market." *Journal of Political Economy* 120 (4): 659–95.

CLARKE, ADELE E.

1998   *Disciplining Reproduction: Modernity, American Life Sciences, and "the Problems of Sex."* Berkeley and Los Angeles: University of California Press.

CLARKE, ADELE E., AND VIRGINIA L. OLESEN, EDS.

1999   *Revisioning Women, Health, and Healing: Feminist, Cultural, and Technoscience Perspectives.* New York: Routledge.

COLE, JOHNNETTA B., AND BEVERLY GUY-SHEFTALL

2003   *Gender Talk: The Struggle for Women's Equality in African American Communities.* New York: One World/Ballantine Books.

COLLINS, PATRICIA HILL

1998a   "It's All in the Family: Intersections of Gender, Race, and Nation." *Hypatia* 13 (3): 62–82.

1998b   "Will the 'Real' Mother Please Stand Up? The Logic of Eugenics and American National Family Planning." In *Revisioning Women, Health, and Healing: Feminist, Cultural, and Technoscience Perspectives*, edited by Adele E. Clarke and Virginia Olesen, 266–82. New York: Routledge.

2004   *Black Sexual Politics: African Americans, Gender, and the New Racism.* New York: Routledge.

COLLS, RACHEL, AND BETHAN EVANS

2009   "Introduction: Questioning Obesity Politics." *Antipode* 41 (5): 1011–20.

CONNELL, ROBERT W.

1995   *Masculinities.* Berkeley and Los Angeles: University of California Press.

CORREA, ADOLFO, AND JESSICA MARCINKEVAGE

2013   "Prepregnancy Obesity and the Risk of Birth Defects: An Update." *Nutrition Reviews* 71 (Suppl. 1): S68–S77.

COUNIHAN, CAROLE

1999   *The Anthropology of Food and Body: Gender, Meaning, and Power.* New York: Routledge.

COYNE, TERRY

2000   *Lifestyle Diseases in Pacific Communities.* Noumea, New Caledonia: Secretariat of the Pacific Community.

CRABTREE, SARA A.

2007   "Culture, Gender and the influence of Social Change amongst Emirati Families in the United Arab Emirates." *Journal of Comparative Family Studies* 38 (4): 575.

CRAWFORD, ROBERT.

1980   "Healthism and the Medicalization of Everyday Life." *International Journal of Health Services* 10 (3): 365–88.

1984   "A Cultural Account of 'Health': Control, Release, and the Social Body." In *Issues in the Political Economy of Health Care,* edited by John McKinlay, 61–103. London: Tavistock.

CRUNK FEMINIST COLLECTIVE

2011   "Slutwalks vs. Ho Strolls." Crunk Feminist Collective, http://www.crunk feministcollective.com/2011/05/23/slutwalks-v-ho-strolls. Accessed June 11, 2015.

DAHL, MELISSA

2013   "'Fat Shaming' Actually Increases Risk of Becoming or Staying Obese, New Study Says." NBC News, July 26. http://www.nbcnews.com/health/diet -fitness/fat-shaming-actually-increases-risk-becoming-or-staying-obese -new-f8C10751491.

DALTON, A., AND S. CROWLEY

2000   "Economic Impact of NCD in the Pacific Islands (with Special Reference to Obesity)." In *Proceedings of the Workshop on Obesity Prevention and Control Strategies in the Pacific, Apia, Western Samoa.* Apia, Western Samoa.

DARMON, NICOLE, AND ADAM DREWNOWSKI

2008   "Does Social Class Predict Diet Quality?" *American Journal of Clinical Nutrition* 87 (5): 1107–17.

DAVID, RICHARD, AND JAMES COLLINS JR.

2007   "Disparities in Infant Mortality: What's Genetics Got to Do with It?" *American Journal of Public Health* 97 (7): 1191–97.

DAVIDSON, CHRISTOPHER

2008   *Dubai: The Vulnerability of Success.* New York: Columbia University Press.

2009   *Abu Dhabi: Oil and Beyond.* New York: Columbia University Press.

DESJARLAIS, ROBERT R.

1992   *Body and Emotion: The Aesthetics of Illness and Healing in the Nepal Himalayas.* Philadelphia: University of Pennsylvania Press.

DESMOND, SHARON M., JAMES H. PRICE, CHRISTOPHER HALLINAN, AND DAISY SMITH

1989   "Black and White Adolescents' Perceptions of Their Weight." *Journal of School Health* 59 (8): 353–58.

DESROSIÈRES, ALAIN

2002   *The Politics of Large Numbers: A History of Statistical Reasoning.* Cambridge: Harvard University Press.

DIAMOND, IRENE, AND LEE QUINBY, EDS.

1988   *Feminism and Foucault: Reflections on Resistance.* Boston: Northeastern University Press.

DICKINS, M., SAMANTHA L. THOMAS, BRI KING, SOPHIE LEWIS, AND KATE HOLLAND

2011   "The Role of the Fatosphere in Fat Adults' Responses to Obesity Stigma: A Model of Empowerment without a Focus on Weight Loss." *Qualitative Health Research* 21 (12): 1679–91.

DINSA, G. D., Y. GORYAKIN, E. FUMAGALLI, AND M. SUHRCKE

2012   "Obesity and Socioeconomic Status in Developing Countries: A Systematic Review." *Obesity Reviews* 11 (13): 1067–79.

DOBBS, RICHARD, AND CORINNE SAWERS

2014   "Obesity: A Global Economic Issue." VOX, CEPR'S Policy Portal. http://voxeu.org/article/obesity-global-economic-issue.

DREWNOWSKI, A.

2009   "Obesity, Diets, and Social Inequalities." *Nutrition Reviews* 67:S36–S39.

DREWNOWSKI, A., AND N. DARMON

2005   "The Economics of Obesity: Dietary Energy Density and Energy Cost." *American Journal of Clinical Nutrition* 82 (1): 265S–273S.

DREWNOWSKI, A., AND S. E. SPECTER

2004   "Poverty and Obesity: The Role of Energy Density and Energy Costs." *American Journal of Clinical Nutrition* 79 (1): 6–16.

DUARTE, NATALIA L., STEPHEN COLAGIURI, TANIELA PALU, XING L. WANG, AND DAVID E. L. WILCHEN

2003   "Obesity, Type II Diabetes and the Beta 2 Adrenoceptor Gene Gln27Glu Polymorphism in the Tongan Population." *Clinical Science* 104:211–15.

DU BOIS, W. E. B.

1994   *The Souls of Black Folk.* Unabridged ed. New York: Dover Publications.

EATON, S. B., M. KONNER, AND M. SHOSTAK

1988   "Stone Agers in the Fast Lane: Chronic Degenerative Diseases in Evolutionary Perspective." *American Journal of Medicine* 84 (4): 739–49.

ECKERT, PENELOPE

1993   "Cooperative Competition in Adolescent 'Girl Talk.'" In *Gender and Conversational Interaction*, edited by Deborah Tannen, 32–61. New York: Oxford University Press.

ECKERT, PENELOPE, AND SALLY MCCONNELL-GINET

1995   "Constructing Meaning, Constructing Selves: Snapshots of Language, Gender, and Class from Belten High." In *Gender Articulated: Language and the Socially Constructed Self*, edited by Kira Hall and Mary Bucholtz, 469–507. New York: Routledge.

ECTOFF, NANCY

1999   *Survival of the Prettiest: The Science of Beauty.* New York: Doubleday.

EDER, DONNA, WITH CATHERINE COLLEEN EVANS AND STEPHEN PARKER

1995   *School Talk: Gender and Adolescent Culture.* New Brunswick, NJ: Rutgers
            University Press.

EDMONDS, ALEXANDER

2010   *Pretty Modern: Beauty, Sex, and Plastic Surgery in Brazil.* Durham, NC: Duke
            University Press.

2012   "Body Image in Non-Western Societies." In *The Encyclopedia of Body Image
            and Human Appearance,* edited by T. Cash, 238–42. New York: Academic
            Press.

2013   "Can Medicine Be Aesthetic? Disentangling Beauty and Health in Elective
            Surgeries." *Medical Anthropology Quarterly* 27 (2): 233–52.

2014   "Surgery-for-Life: Aging, Sexual Fitness and Self-Management in Brazil."
            Anthropology & Aging Quarterly 34 (4): 246–59.

EDMONDS, ALEXANDER, AND EMILIA SANABRIA

2014   "Medical Borderlands: Engineering the Body with Plastic Surgery and Hor-
            monal Therapies in Brazil." *Anthropology & Medicine* 21 (2): 202–16.

EDMONDSON, AIMEE

2005   "Special Report: Infant Mortality in Memphis." *Commercial Appeal,*
            March 6. http://www.commercialappeal.com/news/2005/mar/06
            /special-report-infant-mortality-in-memphis.

EHRENREICH, BARBARA, AND DEIRDRE ENGLISH

1978   *For Her Own Good: Two Centuries of the Experts' Advice to Women.*
            New York: Anchor Books/Doubleday.

EISENBERG, MARLA, DIANNE NEUMARK-SZTAINER, AND MARY STORY

2003   "Associations of Weight-Based Teasing and Emotional Well-Being among
            Adolescents." *Archives of Pediatrics & Adolescent Medicine* 157:733–38.

EISENSTEIN, ZILLAH

n.d.   "Urgent Articulations." Manuscript in progress.

EL-GUINDI, FADWA

1999   *Veil: Modesty, Privacy and Resistance.* New York: Berg.

EL-SAYED, ABDULRAHMAN, PETER SCARBOROUGH, AND SANDRO GALEA

2012   "Unevenly Distributed: A Systematic Review of the Health Literature about
            Socioeconomic Inequalities in Adult Obesity in the United Kingdom." *BMC
            Public Health* 12:18.

FALLON, APRIL

1990   "Culture in the Mirror: Sociocultural Determinants of Body Image." In *Body*

Images: Development, Deviance, and Change, edited by T. F. Cash and T. Pruzinsky, 80–110. New York: Guilford.

FARRELL, AMY E.

2011   *Fat Shame: Stigma and the Fat Body in American Culture.* New York: New York University Press.

FARRER, JAMES

2010   "A Foreign Adventurer's Paradise? Interracial Sexuality and Alien Sexual Capital in Reform Era Shanghai." *Sexualities* 13:69–95.

FAUSTO-STERLING, ANNE

2008   "The Bare Bones of Race." *Social Studies of Science* 38 (5): 657–94.

FEATHERSTONE, MIKE

1982   "The Body in Consumer Culture." *Theory, Culture & Society* 1 (2): 18–33.

FERNEA, ELIZABETH

1965   *Guests of the Sheikh: An Ethnography of an Iraqi Village.* New York: Anchor Books.

FIELD, ALISON E., WITH CARLOS A. CAMARGO AND SHUJI OGINO

2013   "The Merits of Subtyping Obesity: One Size Does Not Fit All." *Journal of the American Medical Association* 310 (20): 2147–48.

FINKELSTEIN, ERIC, OLGA KHAVIOU, HOPE THOMPSON, JUSTIN TROGDON, LIPING PAN, BETTYLOU SHERRY, AND WILLIAM DIETZ

2012   "Obesity and Severe Obesity Forecasts through 2030." *American Journal of Preventative Medicine* 42 (6): 563–70.

FIRTH, JEANNE

2010   "Healthy Choices and Heavy Burdens: Race, Citizenship and Gender in the 'Obesity Epidemic.'" *Journal of International Women's Studies* 13 (2): 33–50.

FLAVIN, JEANNE

2009   *Our Bodies, Our Crimes: The Policing of Women's Reproduction in America.* New York: New York University Press.

FLEGAL, KATHERINE M.

1999   "The Obesity Epidemic in Children and Adults: Current Evidence and Research Issues." *Medicine & Science in Sports & Exercise* 31:S509–S514.

FLEGAL, KATHERINE M., MARGARET D. CARROLL, BRIAN K. KIT, AND CYNTHIA L. OGDEN

2012   "Prevalence of Obesity and Trends in the Distribution of Body Mass Index among US Adults, 1999–2010." *Journal of the American Medical Association* 307 (5): 491–97.

FLEGAL, KATHERINE M., MARGARET D. CARROLL, CYNTHIA L. OGDEN, AND
LESTER R. CURTIN
2010   "Prevalence and Trends in Obesity among United States Adults, 1999–2008."
        Journal of the American Medical Association 303 (3): 235–41.

FLOWERS, KELCI C., MAURICE J. LEVESQUE, AND SARAH FISCHER
2012   "The Relationship between Maladaptive Eating Behaviors and Racial Identity
        among African American Women in College." *Journal of Black Psychology* 38
        (3): 290–312.

FORDE, IAN, T. CHANDOLA, S. GARCIA, M. G. MARMOT, AND O. ATTANASIO
2011   "The Impact of Cash Transfers to Poor Women in Colombia on BMI and
        Obesity: Prospective Cohort Study." *International Journal of Obesity* 36 (9):
        1209–14.

FORDHAM, SIGNITHIA
2008   "Beyond Capital High: On Dual Citizenship and the Strange Career of 'Act-
        ing White.'" *Anthropology & Education Quarterly* 39 (3): 227–46.

FORDYCE, LAUREN
2013   "Accounting for Fetal Death: Vital Statistics and the Medicalization of Preg-
        nancy in the United States." *Social Science and Medicine* 92:124–31.

FOUCAULT, MICHEL
1973   *The Birth of the Clinic: An Archaeology of Medical Perception.* Translated by
        Alan Sheridan. New York: Tavistock.

1977   *Discipline and Punish: The Birth of the Prison.* Translated by Alan Sheridan.
        New York: Pantheon Books.

1990 [1976]   *An Introduction.* Vol. 1 of *The History of Sexuality.* Translated by Robert
        Hurley. New York: Vintage.

1995 [1975]   *Discipline and Punish: The Birth of the Prison.* Translated by Alan Sheri-
        dan. 2nd ed. New York: Vintage.

2010   *The Birth of Biopolitics: Lectures at the Collège de France, 1978–1979.* New
        York: Picador.

FRANKLIN, DEBORAH
2006   "Can a Baby Be Too Fat?" NPR, November 2. http://www.npr.org/templates
        /story/story.php?storyId=6417869.

FREDA, MARGARET COMERFORD, MERRY-K. MOOS, AND MICHELE CURTIS
2006   "The History of Preconception Care: Evolving Guidelines and Standards."
        Maternal and Child Health Journal 10:S43–S52.

FREEDMAN, DAVID H.
2011   "How to Fix the Obesity Crisis." *Scientific American*, February. http://www
        .scientificamerican.com/article/how-to-fix-the-obesity-crisis.

FREEDMAN, RACHEL E. K., MICHELE M. CARTER, TRACY SBROCCO, AND JAMES J. GRAY
2004 "Ethnic Differences in Preferences for Female Weight and Waist-to-Hip Ratio: A Comparison of African-American and White American College and Community Samples." *Eating Behaviors* 5 (3): 191–98.

FREEMAN, DILYS J.
2010 "Effects of Maternal Obesity on Fetal Growth and Body Composition: Implications for Programming and Future Health." *Seminars in Fetal and Neonatal Medicine* 15:113–18.

FRIEDMAN, JEFFREY M.
2004 "Modern Science versus the Stigma of Obesity." *Nature Medicine* 10:563–69.

FRIEDMAN, K. E., S. K. REICHMANN, P. R. COSTANZO, ET AL.
2005 "Weight Stigmatization and Ideological Beliefs: Relation to Psychological Functioning in Obese Adults." *Obesity Research* 13:907–16.

GARD, MICHAEL
2010 "Truth, Belief and the Cultural Politics of Obesity Scholarship and Public Health Policy." *Critical Public Health* 21 (1): 37–48.

GARNER, DAVID M., PAUL E. GARFINKEL, DONALD SCHWARTZ, AND
MICHAEL THOMPSON
1980 "Cultural Expectations of Thinness in Women." *Psychological Reports* 47:483–91.

GARRETT, EILIDH, CHRIS GALLEY, NICOLA SHELTON, AND ROBERT WOODS
2007 *Infant Mortality: A Continuing Social Problem.* Aldershot, UK: Ashgate.

GASKIN, DARRELL J., ALVIN E. HEADEN, AND SHELLEY I. WHITE-MEANS
2005 "Racial Disparities in Health and Wealth: The Effects of Slavery and Past Discrimination." *Review of Black Political Economy* 32 (3/4): 95–110.

GERBASI, MARGARET E., LAUREN K. RICHARDS, JENNIFER J. THOMAS,
JESSICA C. AGNEW-BLAIS, HEATHER THOMPSON-BRENNER, STEPHEN E. GILMAN,
AND ANNE E. BECKER
2014 "Globalization and Eating Disorder Risk: Peer Influence, Perceived Social Norms, and Adolescent Disordered Eating in Fiji." *International Journal of Eating Disorders* 47 (7): 727–37.

GERBENSKY-KERBER, ANNE
2011 "Grading the 'Good' Body: A Poststructuralist Feminist Analysis of Body Mass Index Initiatives." *Health Communication* 26 (4): 354–65.

GERBER, LYNNE, AND SARAH QUINN
2008 "Blue Chip Bodies, Fat Phobia, and the Cultural Economy of Body Size." In *Bodily Inscriptions: Interdisciplinary Explorations into Embodiment*, edited by L. D. Kelly, 1–26. Newcastle, UK: Cambridge Scholars.

GHANNAM, FARHA

1997   *Fertile, Plump, and Strong: The Social Construction of the Female Body in Low-Income Cairo.* Monographs in Reproductive Health 3. Cairo: Population Council.

GIDDENS, ANTHONY

1991   *Modernity and Self-Identity.* Stanford, CA: Stanford University Press.

1993   *The Transformation of Intimacy: Sexuality, Love, and Eroticism in Modern Societies.* Stanford, CA: Stanford University Press.

GILL, ROSALIND, KAREN HENWOOD, AND CARL MCLEAN

2005   "Body Projects and the Regulation of Normative Masculinity." *Body & Society* 11 (1): 37–62.

GILLIGAN, CAROL

1993 [1982]   *In a Different Voice: Psychological Theory and Women's Development.* Reissue ed. Cambridge: Harvard University Press.

2011   *Joining the Resistance.* Malden, MA: Polity Press.

GILLMAN, MATTHEW W., AND LUCILLA POSTON, EDS.

2012   *Maternal Obesity.* Cambridge: Cambridge University Press.

GIMLIN, DEBRA

2002   *Body Work: Beauty and Self-Image in American Culture.* Berkeley and Los Angeles: University of California Press.

2007   "What Is Body Work? A Review of the Literature." *Sociology Compass* 1 (1): 353–70.

GOFFMAN, ERVING

1959   *The Presentation of Self in Everyday Life.* New York: Doubleday/Anchor.

1963   *Stigma: Notes on the Management of Spoiled Identity.* New York: Simon & Schuster.

1976   "Gender Advertisements." *Studies in the Anthropology of Visual Communication* 3 (2): 69–154.

GOLDENBERG, MIRIAN

2000   "De Amelias a Operarias: Um Ensaio sobre os Conflitos Femininos no Mercado de Trabalho e nas Relações Conjugais." In *Os novos desejos*, edited by M. Goldenberg. Rio de Janeiro: Record.

GORDON-LARSEN, PENNY, MELISSA C. NELSON, PHIL PAGE, AND BARRY M. POPKIN

2006   "Inequality in the Built Environment Underlies Key Health Disparities in Physical Activity and Obesity." *Pediatrics* 117 (2): 417–24.

GORTMAKER, STEVEN L., AVIVA MUST, JAMES M. PERRIN, ARTHUR M. SOBOL, AND
WILLIAM H. DIETZ

1993   "Social and Economic Consequences of Overweight in Adolescence and
        Young Adulthood." *New England Journal of Medicine* 329 (14): 1008–12.

GRABE, SHELLY, AND JANET SHIBLEY HYDE

2006   "Ethnicity and Body Dissatisfaction among Women in the United States:
        A Meta-analysis." *Psychological Bulletin* 132 (4): 622–40.

GRANBERG, ELLEN M., RONALD L. SIMONS, FREDERICK X. GIBBONS, AND
JANET N. MELBY

2008   "The Relationship between Body Size and Depressed Mood: Findings from
        a Sample of African American Middle School Girls." *Youth & Society* 39 (3):
        294–315.

GRAZIAN, DAVID

2008   *On the Make: The Hustle of Urban Nightlife.* Chicago: University of Chicago
        Press.

GREEN, ADAM I.

2011   "Playing the (Sexual) Field: The Interactional Basis of Systems of Sexual
        Stratification." *Social Psychology Quarterly* 74 (3): 244–66.

2013   "'Erotic Capital' and the Power of Desirability: Why 'Honey Money' Is a Bad
        Collective Strategy for Remedying Gender Inequality." *Sexualities* 16:137–58.

GREENBERG, DEBORAH R., AND DAVID J. LAPORTE

1996   "Racial Differences in Body Type Preferences of Men and Women." *Interna-
        tional Journal of Eating Disorders* 19:275–78.

GREENHALGH, SUSAN

2015   *Fat-Talk Nation: The Human Costs of America's War on Fat.* Ithaca, NY:
        Cornell University Press.

GREENHALGH, SUSAN, AND MEGAN CARNEY

2014   "Bad Biocitizens? Latinos and the U.S. 'Obesity Epidemic.'" *Human Organi-
        zation* 73 (3): 267–76.

GREMILLION, HELEN

2005   "The Cultural Politics of Body Size." *Annual Reviews in Anthropology* 34:
        13–32.

GRIFFITHS, LUCY, AND ANGIE PAGE

2008   "The Impact of Weight-Related Victimization on Peer Relationships: The
        Female Adolescent Perspective." *Obesity* 16 (Suppl. 2): S39–S44.

GROGAN, SARAH

2007   *Body Image: Understanding Body Dissatisfaction in Men, Women and Chil-
        dren.* New York: Routledge.

GROGAN, SARAH, AND HELEN RICHARDS

2002   "Body Image: Focus Groups with Boys and Men." *Men and Masculinities* 4 (3): 219–32.

GRØNNING, INGEBORG, GRAHAM SCAMBLER, AND AKSEL TJORA

2013   "From Fatness to Badness: The Modern Morality of Obesity." *Health* 17 (3): 266–83.

Guthman, Julie

2012   "Doing Justice to Bodies? Reflections on Food Justice, Race, and Biology." *Antipode* 46 (5): 1153–71.

HADLEY, CRAIG, AND D. J. HRUSCHKA

2014   "Population Level Differences in Adult Body Mass Emerge in Infancy and Early Childhood: Evidence from a Global Sample of Low and Lower-Income Countries." *American Journal of Physical Anthropology* 154 (2): 232–38.

HAKIM, CATHERINE

2010   "Erotic Capital." *European Sociological Review* 26:499–518.

HAMMERMESH, DANIEL

2011   *Beauty Pays: Why Attractive People Are More Successful.* Princeton, NJ: Princeton University Press.

HAN, EUNA, EDWARD C. NORTON, AND LISA M. POWELL

2011   "Direct and Indirect Effects of Body Weight on Adult Wages." *Economics & Human Biology* 9 (4): 381–92.

HAN, EUNA, EDWARD C. NORTON, AND SALLY C. STEARNS

2009   "Weight and Wages: Fat versus Lean Paychecks." *Health Economics* 18 (5): 535–48.

HAN, Z., S. MULLA, J. BEYENE, G. LIAO, S. D. MCDONALD, AND
KNOWLEDGE SYNTHESIS GROUP

2011   "Maternal Underweight and the Risk of Preterm Birth and Low Birth Weight: A Systematic Review and Meta-Analyses." *International Journal of Epidemiology* 40 (1): 65–101.

HANSEN, JANET

2014   "Explode and Die! A Fat Women's Perspective on Prenatal Care and the Fat Panic Epidemic." *Narrative Enquiry in Bioethics* 4 (2): 99–101.

HARAWAY, DONNA

1985   "Manifesto for Cyborgs: Science, Technology, and Socialist Feminism in the 1980s." *Socialist Review* 80:65–108.

HARPER, BARRY

2000   "Beauty, Stature and the Labour Market: A British Cohort Study." *Oxford Bulletin of Economics and Statistics* 62 (s1): 771–800.

HARRIS, SHANETTE M.

1995   "Family, Self and Sociocultural Contributions to Body-Image Attitudes of African-American Women." *Psychology of Women Quarterly* 19 (1): 129–45.

HASSO, FRANCES

2011   *Consuming Desires: Family Crisis and the State in the Middle East.* Stanford, CA: Stanford University Press.

HEALTH AUTHORITY ABU DHABI (HAAD)

2013   *Health Statistics 2012.* Abu Dhabi, UAE: HAAD Annual Report.

HEARD-BEY, FRAUKE

2004   *From Trucial States to United Arab Emirates: A Society in Transition.* Reprint with a new foreword. Abu Dhabi: Motivate.

HEBL, MICHELLE R., AND LAURA M. MANNIX

2003   "The Weight of Obesity in Evaluating Others: A Mere Proximity Effect." *Personality and Social Psychology Bulletin* 29 (1): 28–38.

HEBL, MIKKI R., AND LAURA M. MANNIX

2003   "The Weight of Obesity in Evaluating Others: A Mere Proximity Effect." *Personality and Social Psychology Bulletin* 29 (1): 28–38.

HERNDON, APRIL MICHELLE

2006   "Collateral Damage from Friendly Fire? Race, Nation, Class and the 'War Against Obesity.'" *Social Semiotics* 15 (2): 127–41.

HESSE-BIBER, SHARLENE N.

1996   *Am I Thin Enough Yet? The Cult of Thinness and the Commercialization of Identity.* Berkeley and Los Angeles: University of California Press.

HILL, SHIRLEY A.

2002   "Teaching and Doing Gender in African American Families." *Sex Roles* 47 (11–12): 493–506.

HODGE, ALLISON M., GARY K. DOWSE, P. TOELUPE, VERONICA R. COLLINS, T. IMO, AND PAUL Z. ZIMMET

1994   "Dramatic Increase in the Prevalence of Obesity in Western Samoa over the 13-Year Period 1978–1991." *International Journal of Obesity and Related Metabolic Disorders* 18 (6): 419–28.

HODGE, ALLISON M., GARY K. DOWSE, PAUL Z. ZIMMET, AND VERONICA R. COLLINS

1995   "Prevalence and Secular Trends in Obesity in Pacific and Indian Ocean Island Populations." *Obesity Research* 3 (S2): 77s–87s.

HOLLIDAY, RUTH, AND JOANNA ELFVING-HWANG

2012   "Gender, Globalization, and Aesthetic Surgery in South Korea." *Body & Society* 18 (2): 58–81.

HOOKS, BELL

1981   *Ain't I a Woman: Black Women and Feminism.* Boston: South End Press.

HRUSCHKA, DANIEL J.

2012   "Do Economic Constraints on Food Choice Make People Fat? A Critical Review of Two Hypotheses for the Poverty-Obesity Paradox." *American Journal of Human Biology* 24 (3): 277–85.

HRUSCHKA, DANIEL, AND ALEXANDRA BREWIS

2013   "Absolute Wealth and World Region Strongly Predict Overweight among Women (Ages 18–49) in 360 Populations across 36 Developing Countries." *Economics & Human Biology* 11 (3): 337–44.

HRUSCHKA, D. J., D. GERKEY, AND CRAIG HADLEY

2015   "Estimating the Absolute Wealth of Households." *Bulletin of the World Health Organization* 93 (7): 483–90.

HRUSCHKA, DANIEL J., CRAIG HADLEY, AND ALEXANDRA BREWIS

2014   "Disentangling Basal and Accumulated Body Mass for Cross-Population Comparisons." *American Journal of Physical Anthropology* 153 (4): 542–50.

HRUSCHKA, D. J., CRAIG HADLEY, ALEXANDRA A. BREWIS, AND CHRISTOPHER M. STOJANOWSKI

2015   "Genetic Population Structure Accounts for Ecogeographic Rules in Tropic and Subtropic Dwelling Humans." *PLOS ONE* 10 (3).

HRUSCHKA, D. J., AND A. HAGAMAN

2015   "The Physiological Cost of Reproduction for Rich and Poor across 65 Countries." *American Journal of Human Biology* 27 (5): 654–59.

HRUSCHKA, D. J., E. C. RUSH, AND A. A. BREWIS

2013   "Population Differences in the Relationship between Height, Weight, and Adiposity: An Application of Burton's Model." *American Journal of Physical Anthropology* 151 (1): 68–76.

HUDSON, JAMES I., EVA HIRIPI, HARRISON G. POPE JR., AND RONALD C. KESSLER

2007   "The Prevalence and Correlates of Eating Disorders in the National Comorbidity Survey Replication." *Biological Psychiatry* 61 (3): 348–58.

HUFF, JOYCE

2001   "A 'Horror of Corpulence': Interrogating Bantingism and Mid-Nineteenth Century Fat-Phobia." In *Bodies Out of Bounds: Fatness and Transgression*, edited by Jana Evans Braziel and Kathleen LeBesco, 39–59. Berkeley and Los Angeles: University of California Press.

ICF MACRO

n.d.   Demographic and Health Surveys. Calverton, MD.

JACOBY, SALLY, AND ELINOR OCHS

1995   "Co-Construction: An Introduction." *Research on Language and Social Interaction* 28 (3): 171–83.

JACKSON, LINDA A.

1992   *Physical Appearance and Gender: Sociobiological and Sociocultural Perspectives.* New York: State University of New York Press.

JACKSON, T., C. GRILO, AND R. MASHEB

2000   "Teasing History, Onset of Obesity, Current Eating Disorder Psychopathology, Body Dissatisfaction, and Psychological Functioning in Binge Eating Disorder." *Obesity Research* 8 (6): 451–58.

JAMES, CARYL

2012   *Dying to Be Beautiful.* Mona, Jamaica: University of the West Indies.

JEHN, MEGAN, AND ALEXANDRA BREWIS

2009   "Paradoxical Malnutrition in Mother-Child Pairs: Untangling the Phenomenon of Over- and Under-Nutrition in Underdeveloped Economies." *Economics and Human Biology* 7:28–35.

JOHNSON, CRAIG L., MARILYN K. STUCKEY, LINDA D. LEWIS, AND DONALD M. SCHWARTZ

1982   "Bulimia: A Descriptive Survey of 316 Cases." *International Journal of Eating Disorders* 2 (1): 3–16.

JOHNSON, KAY A.

2010   "Women's Health and Health Reform: Implications of the Patient Protection and Affordable Care Act." *Current Opinion in Obstetrics and Gynecology* 22 (6): 492–97.

JONES, ARTHUR F., JR., AND DANIEL H. WEINBERG

2000   "The Changing Shape of the Nation's Income Distribution." *Current Population Reports* 60:1–11.

JONES, EDWARD E., AMERIGO FARINA, ALBERT H. HASTORF, HAZEL MARKUS, DALE T. MILLER, AND ROBERT A. SCOTT

1984   *Social Stigma: The Psychology of Marked Relationships.* New York: Freeman.

KARKAZIS, KATRINA

2008   *Fixing Sex: Intersex, Medical Authority, and Lived Experience.* Durham, NC: Duke University Press.

KASSIRER, JEROME P., AND MARCIA ANGELL

1998   "Losing Weight—An Ill-Fated New Year's Resolution." *New England Journal of Medicine* 338 (1): 52.

KATZ, MIRA L., PENNY GORDON-LARSEN, MARGARET E. BENTLEY, KRISTINE KELSEY, KENITRA SHIELDS, AND ALICE AMMERMAN

2004   "'Does Skinny Mean Healthy?' Perceived Ideal, Current, and Healthy Body Sizes Among African-American Girls and Their Female Caregivers." *Ethnicity & Disease* 14 (4): 533–41.

KATZ, STANLEY, AND BARBARA MARSHALL

2003   "New Sex for Old: Lifestyle, Consumerism, and the Ethics of Aging Well."
          Journal of Aging Studies 17 (1): 3–16.

KATZMAN, MELANIE, WITH KARIN M. E. HERMANS, DAPHNE VAN HOEKEN, AND
HANS W. HOEK

2004   "Not Your 'Typical Island Woman': Anorexia Is Reported Only in Subcul-
          tures on Curacao." *Culture, Medicine, and Psychiatry* 28 (4): 463–92.

KAUFMAN, NANCY, AND MIMI NICHTER

2010   "The Marketing of Tobacco to Women: Global Perspectives." In *Gender,
          Women, and the Tobacco Epidemic*, by WHO. Geneva: WHO.

KAW, EUGENIA

1993   "Medicalization of Racial Features: Asian American Women and Cosmetic
          Surgery." *Medical Anthropology Quarterly* 7:74–89.

KEHLER, MICHAEL

2010   "Negotiating Masculinities in PE Classrooms: Boys, Body Image, and 'Want-
          [ing] to Be in Good Shape.'" In *Boys' Bodies: Speaking the Unspoken*, edited
          by Michael Kehler and Michael Atkinson, 153–75. New York: Peter Lang.

KEITH, LOUIS G.

2006   "Is It Time to 'Bang the Shoe' on Preconception Care?" *Maternal and Child
          Health Journal* 10:S1–S2.

KEITH, SCOTT W., WITH DAVID T. REDDEN, PETER KATZMARZYK, MARY BOGGIANO,
ERIN C. HANLON, RUTH M. BENCA, DOUGLAS RUDEN, ANGELO PIETROBELLI, JAMIE L.
BARGER, KEVIN R. FONTAINE, C. WANG, LOUIS J. ARONNE, SCOTT M. WRIGHT,
MONICA L. BASKIN, NIKHIL DHURANDHAR, MARIA C. LIJOI, CARLOS M. GRILO,
MARIA DE LUCA, ANDREW O. WESTFALL, AND DAVID B. ALLISON

2006   "Putative Contributors to the Secular Increase in Obesity: Exploring the
          Roads Less Traveled." *International Journal of Obesity* 30 (11): 1585–94.

KEMP, LINZI J.

2013   "Progress in Female Education and Employment in the United Arab
          Emirates towards Millennium Development Goal (3): Gender Equality."
          Foresight: The Journal of Futures Studies, Strategic Thinking and Policy 15 (4):
          264–77.

KEMP, MATTHEW W., SUHA G. KALLAPUR, ALAN H. JOBE, AND JOHN P. NEWNHAM

2012   "Obesity and the Developmental Origins of Health and Disease." *Journal
          of Pediatrics and Child Health* 48:86–90.

KIRKLAND, ANNA

2011   "The Environmental Account of Obesity: A Case for Feminist Skepticism."
          Signs 36 (2): 463–85.

KOHM, AMELIA

2007   "Embarrassment of the Richest: Reducing Infant Mortality in the U.S."
        Prevention Action, July 25. http://preventionaction.org/what-works
        /embarrassment-richest-reducing-infant-mortality-us.

KUZAWA, C. W., AND E. SWEET.

2009   "Epigenetics and the Embodiment of Race: Developmental Origins of US
        Racial Disparities in Cardiovascular Health." *American Journal of Human
        Biology* 21 (1): 2–15.

KVERNFLATEN, BIRGIT

2013   "Meeting Targets or Saving Lives: Maternal Health Policy and Millennium
        Development Goal 5 in Nicaragua." *Reproductive Health Matters* 21 (42):
        32–40.

KWAN, SAMANTHA

2009   "Individual versus Corporate Responsibility: Market Choice, the Food
        Industry, and the Pervasiveness of Moral Models of Fatness. *Food, Culture,
        & Society* 12 (4): 478–95.

KWAN, SAMANTHA, AND JENNIFER GRAVES

2013   *Framing Fat: Competing Constructions in Contemporary Culture.* New Bruns-
        wick, NJ: Rutgers University Press.

LAMONT, MICHELLE, AND VIRAG MOLNAR

2002   "The Study of Boundaries in the Social Sciences." *Annual Review of Sociology*
        28:167–95.

LASCH, CHRISTOPHER

1979   *The Culture of Narcissism: American Life in an Age of Diminishing Expecta-
        tions.* New York: Warner Books.

LAU, KIMBERLY J.

2011   *Body Language: Sisters in Shape, Black Women's Fitness, and Feminist Identity
        Politics.* Philadelphia: Temple University Press.

LAVEIST, THOMAS A.

2000   "On the Study of Race, Racism, and Health: A Shift from Description to
        Explanation." *International Journal of Health Services* 30 (1): 217–19.

2005   "Disentangling Race and Socioeconomic Status: A Key to Solving Health
        Disparities." *Journal of Urban Health* 82 (2 Suppl. 13): iii26–iii34.

LAWRENCE, REGINA G.

2004   "Framing Obesity: The Evolution of News Discourse on a Public Health
        Issue." *Harvard International Journal of Press/Politics* 9 (3): 56–75.

LEBESCO, KATHLEEN

2011   "Neoliberalism, Public Health, and the Moral Perils of Fatness." *Critical
        Public Health* 21 (2): 153–64.

LEE, SHU-YUEH

2009   "The Power of Beauty in Reality Plastic Surgery Shows: Romance, Career, and Happiness." *Communication, Culture & Critique* 2:503–19.

LE GRANGE, DANIEL, JOHANN LOUW, ALISON BREEN, AND MELANIE A. KATZMAN

2004   "The Meaning of 'Self-Starvation' in Impoverished Black Adolescents in South Africa." *Culture, Medicine, and Psychiatry* 28:439–61.

LEICHTER, HOWARD M.

2003   "'Evil Habits' and 'Personal Choices': Assigning Responsibility for Health in the 20th Century." *Milbank Quarterly* 81 (4): 603–26.

LESTER, REBECCA

1997   "The (Dis)Embodied Self in Anorexia Nervosa." *Social Science and Medicine* 44 (4): 479–89.

LOGAN, TREVOR

2010   "Personal Characteristics, Sexual Behaviors, and Male Sex Work: A Quantitative Approach." *American Sociological Review* 75 (5): 679–704.

LUNNER, KATARINA, ELEANOR H. WERTHEM, JOEL K. THOMPSON, SUSAN J. PAXTON, FIONA MCDONALD, AND KLARA S. HALVAARSON

2000   "A Cross-Cultural Examination of Weight-Related Teasing, Body Image, and Eating Disturbance in Swedish and Australian Samples." *International Journal of Eating Disorders* 28 (4): 430–35.

LUPPINO, FLORIANA S., LEONORE M. DE WIT, PAUL F. BOUVY, THEO STIJNEN, PIM CUIJPERS, BRENDA W. J. H. PENNINX, AND FRANS G. ZITMAN

2010   "Overweight, Obesity, and Depression: A Systematic Review and Meta-Analysis of Longitudinal Studies." *Archives of General Psychiatry* 67 (3): 220–29.

MACKENZIE, MARGARET

1985   "The Pursuit of Slenderness and Addiction to Self-Control." In *Nutrition Update*, vol. 2, edited by Jean Weininger and George M. Briggs, 174–94. New York: John Wiley and Sons.

MACLEAN, LYNNE, NANCY EDWARDS, MICHAEL GARRARD, NICKI SIMS-JONES, KATHRYN CLINTON, AND LISA ASHLEY

2009   "Obesity, Stigma, and Public Health Planning." *Health Promotion International* 24 (1): 88–93.

MADDOX, GEORGE L., KURT W. BACK, AND VERONICA R. LIEDERMAN

1968   "Overweight as Social Deviance and Disability." *Journal of Health and Social Behavior* 9 (4): 287–300.

MAHMOOD, SABA

2005   *Politics of Piety: The Islamic Revival and the Feminist Project.* Princeton, NJ: Princeton University Press.

MARCUS, MARSHA D., AND JENNIFER E. WILDES
2009   "Obesity: Is It a Mental Disorder?" *International Journal of Eating Disorders*
        42 (8): 739–53.

MARTIN, DANIEL
2010   "Obese? Just Call Them Fat: Plain-Speaking Doctors Will Jolt People into
        Losing Weight, Says Minister." *Daily Mail*, July 29. http://www.dailymail
        .co.uk/news/article-1298394/Call-overweight-people-fat-instead-obese-says
        -health-minister.html. Accessed March 6, 2015.

MARTIN, JOHN LEVI, AND MATT GEORGE
2006   "Theories of Sexual Stratification: Toward an Analytics of the Sexual Field
        and a Theory of Sexual Capital." *Sociological Theory* 24 (2): 107–32.

MATHEWS, T. J., AND MARIAN MACDORMAN
2011   "Infant Mortality Statistics from the 2007 Period Linked Birth/Infant Death
        Data Set." *National Vital Statistics Reports* 59, no 6.

MAVOA, HELEN M., AND MARITA MCCABE
2008   "Sociocultural Factors Relating to Tongans' and Indigenous Fijians' Patterns
        of Eating, Physical Activity and Body Size." *Asia Pacific Journal of Clinical
        Nutrition* 17 (3): 375–84.

MBEMBE, ACHILLE
2003   "Necropolitics." *Public Culture* 15 (1): 11–40.

MCCLAM, ERIN
2007   "A City's Grief: Memphis' Infant Death Epidemic." NBC News, November 11.
        http://www.nbcnews.com/id/21655131/#.Uu04_nddXzg.

MCCLURE, STEPHANIE
2013   "'It's Just Gym': Physicality and Identity among African American Adoles-
        cent Girls." PhD diss., Case Western Reserve University.

MCCLURE, STEPHANIE, MAURITA POOLE, AND EILEEN P. ANDERSON-FYE
2012   "Race, Ethnicity, and Human Appearance." In *Encyclopedia of Body Image
        and Human Appearance*, edited by Thomas F. Cash, 707–10. New York: Aca-
        demic Press.

MCGARVEY, STEPHEN T.
1991   "Obesity in Samoans and a Perspective on Its Etiology in Polynesians."
        American Journal of Clinical Nutrition 53 (6 Suppl.): 1586s–1594s.

MCGUIRE, W., L. DYSON, AND M. RENFREW
2009   "Maternal Obesity: Consequences for Children, Challenges for Clinicians
        and Carers." *Seminars in Fetal and Neonatal Medicine* 15:108–12.

MCLAREN, MARGARET
2002   *Feminism, Foucault, and Embodied Subjectivity*. New York: State University
        of New York Press.

MCNAUGHTON, DARLENE

2011   "From the Womb to the Tomb: Obesity and Maternal Responsibility."
          Critical Public Health 21 (2): 179–90.

MEARS, ASHLEY

2011   *Pricing Beauty: The Making of a Fashion Model.* Berkeley and Los Angeles:
          University of California Press.

2014   "Who Runs the Girls?" Op-ed. *New York Times Sunday Review,*
          September 21.

MEERA, MARTA, AND LINDSEY RICCARDI

2008   *Obesity Surgery: Stores of Altered Lives.* Las Vegas: University of Nevada
          Press.

MENDELSON, B. K., L. MCLAREN, L. GAUVIN, AND H. STEIGER

2002   "The Relationship of Self-Esteem and Body Esteem in Women with and
          without Eating Disorders." *International Journal of Eating Disorders* 31:
          318–23.

METCALF, PATRICIA A., ROBERT K. R. SCRAGG, P. WILLOUGHBY, SITALEKI A. FINAU,
AND DAVID TIPENE-LEACH

2000   "Ethnic Differences in Perceptions of Body Size in Middle-Aged European,
          Maori and Pacific People Living in New Zealand." *International Journal of
          Obesity and Related Metabolic Disorders* 24:593–99.

MILLER, GREGORY E., EDITH CHEN, AND GENE H. BRODY

2014   "Can Upward Mobility Cost You Your Health?" *New York Times,* January 4.
          http://opinionator.blogs.nytimes.com/2014/01/04/can-upward-mobility
          -cost-you-your-health.

MILLER, LAURA

2006   *Beauty Up: Exploring Contemporary Japanese Body Aesthetics.* Berkeley and
          Los Angeles: University of California Press.

MILLMAN, MARCIA

1980   *Such a Pretty Face: Being Fat in America.* New York: W. W. Norton.

MONK, ELLIS, JR.

2014   "Skin Tone Stratification among Black Americans, 2001–2003." *Social Forces*
          92 (4): 1313–37.

MONTEIRO, C. A., W. L. CONDE, B. LU, AND B. M. POPKIN

2004   "Obesity and Inequities in Health in the Developing World." *International
          Journal of Obesity* 28:1181–86.

MOORE, LISA JEAN, AND MONICA J. CASPER

2014   *The Body: Social and Cultural Dissections.* London: Routledge.

MORRIS, THERESA

2013   *Cut It Out: The C-Section Epidemic in America.* New York: New York University Press.

MORTON, PATRICIA

1991   *Disfigured Images: The Historical Assault on Afro-American Women.* Westport, CT: Greenwood.

MUKHOPADHYAY, SANKAR

2008   "Do Women Value Marriage More? The Effect of Obesity on Cohabitation and Marriage in the USA." *Review of Economics of the Household* 6 (2): 111–26.

MULVEY, LAURA

1975   "Visual Pleasure and Narrative Cinema." *Screen* 16 (3): 6–18.

MURRAY, CHRISTOPHER J. L., THEO VOS, RAFAEL LOZANO, ET AL.

2012   "Disability-Adjusted Life Years (DALYs) for 291 Diseases and Injuries in 21 Regions, 1990–2010: A Systematic Analysis for the Global Burden of Disease Study 2010." *Lancet* 380 (9859): 2197–223.

MURTAGH, LINDSEY, AND DAVID S. LUDWIG

2011   "State Intervention in Life-Threatening Childhood Obesity." *Journal of the American Medical Association* 306 (2): 206–7.

NATIONAL CENTER FOR HEALTH STATISTICS (NCHS)

2014   "Healthy People 2020 Progress Review: Nutrition and Weight Status, and Physical Activity." National Center for Health Statistics, May 9. http://www.cdc.gov/nchs/healthy_people/hp2020/hp2020_NWS_HP_progress_review.htm. Accessed March 3, 2015.

NATIONAL FOOD AND NUTRITION CENTRE

2007   *2004 Fiji National Nutrition Survey—Main Report.* Suva, Fiji: National Food and Nutrition Centre.

NATIONAL HEALTH AND NUTRITION EXAMINATION SURVEY (NHANES)

2011   *Demographics and Examination.* Hyattsville, MD: Department of Health and Human Services, Centers for Disease Control and Prevention.

NAVARRO, VICENTE

1993   *Dangerous to Your Health: Capitalism in Health Care.* New York: Monthly Review Press.

NEUMARK-SZTAINER, DIANNE, MARY STORY, AND LOREN FAIBISCH

1998   "Perceived Stigmatization among Overweight African American and Caucasian Adolescent Girls." *Journal of Adolescent Health* 23:264–70.

NEWMAN, GEORGE

1906   *Infant Mortality: A Social Problem.* London: Methuen.

NG, M., T. FLEMING, M. ROBINSON, ET AL.

2014   "Global, Regional, and National Prevalence of Overweight and Obesity in Children and Adults during 1980–2013: A Systematic Analysis for the Global Burden of Disease Study 2013." *Lancet* 384:766–81.

NICHTER, MARK, AND MIMI NICHTER

1991   "Hype and Weight." *Medical Anthropology* 13 (3): 249–84.

NICHTER, MIMI

2000   *Fat Talk: What Girls and Their Parents Say about Dieting.* Cambridge: Harvard University Press.

NICKSON, DENNIS, CHRIS WARHURST, ANNE WITZ, AND ANNE MARIE CULLEN

2001   "The Importance of Being Aesthetic: Work, Employment and Service Organization." In *Customer Service*, edited by A. Sturdy, I. Grugulis, and H. Willmott. Basingstoke, UK: Palgrave.

OAKS, LAURY

2001   *Smoking and Pregnancy: The Politics of Fetal Protection.* New Brunswick, NJ: Rutgers University Press.

OGDEN, CYNTHIA L., MARGARET D. CARROLL, LESTER R. CURTIN, MARGARET A. MCDOWELL, CAROLYN J. TABAK, AND KATHERINE M. FLEGAL

2006   "Prevalence of Overweight and Obesity in the United States, 1999–2004." *Journal of the American Medical Association* 295 (13): 1549–55.

OGDEN, JANE, AND CECELIA CLEMENTI

2010   "The Experience of Being Obese and the Many Consequences of Stigma." *Journal of Obesity.* http://dx.doi.org/10.1155/2010/429098. Accessed May 2015.

OMI, MICHAEL, AND HOWARD WINANT

1986   *Racial Formation in the United States: From the 1960s to the 1980s.* New York: Routledge and Kegan Paul.

O'NEILL, SHANNON K.

2003   "African American Women and Eating Disturbances: A Meta-Analysis." *Journal of Black Psychology* 29 (1): 3–16.

OPOLINER, APRIL, DEBORAH BLACKER, GARRET FITZMAURICE, AND ANNE BECKER

2013   "Challenges in Assessing Depressive Symptoms in Fiji: A Psychometric Evaluation of the CES-D." *International Journal of Social Psychiatry* 60 (4): 367–76.

ORBACH, SUSIA

1978   *Fat Is a Feminist Issue.* New York: Arrow.

OREFFICE, SONIA, AND CLIMENT QUINTANA-DOMEQUE

2010   "Anthropometry and Socioeconomics among Couples: Evidence in the United States." *Economics & Human Biology* 8 (3): 373–84.

OSBURG, JOHN

2013   *Anxious Wealth: Money and Morality among China's New Rich.* Stanford, CA: Stanford University Press.

OSTERMAN, MICHELLE J. K., JOYCE A. MARTIN, SALLY C. CURTIN, T. J. MATHEWS, ELIZABETH C. WILSON, AND SHARON KIRMEYER

2013   "Newly Released Data from the Revised U.S. Birth Certificate, 2011." *National Vital Statistics Report* 62 (4): 1–22.

OUSLEY, LOUISE, ELIZABETH D. CORDERO, AND SABINA WHITE

2008   "Fat Talk among College Students: How Undergraduates Communicate Regarding Food and Body Weight, Shape and Appearance." *Eating Disorders* 16 (1): 73–84.

PACE, GINA

2006   "Obesity Bigger Threat than Terrorism?" CBS News, March 1. http://www.cbsnews.com/2100-204_162-1361849.html. Accessed March 2, 2015.

PALTROW, LYNN M., AND JEANNE FLAVIN

2013   "Arrests of and Forced Interventions on Pregnant Women in the United States, 1973–2005: Implications for Women's Legal Status and Public Health." *Journal of Health Politics, Policy and Law* 38 (2): 299–343.

PAN, JAY, XUEZHENG QIN, AND GORDON G. LIU

2012   "The Impact of Body Size on Urban Employment: Evidence from China." *China Economic Review* 27:249–63.

PARENS, ERIK, ED.

2006   *Surgically Shaping Children: Technology, Ethics, and the Pursuit of Normality.* Baltimore: Johns Hopkins University Press.

PARKER, RICHARD, AND PETER AGGLETON

2003   "HIV and AIDS-Related Stigma and Discrimination: A Conceptual Framework and Implications for Action." *Social Science and Medicine* 57 (1): 13–24.

PARKER, SHEILA, MIMI NICHTER, MARK NICHTER, NANCY VUCKOVIC, COLETTE SIMS, AND CHERYL RITENBAUGH

1995   "Body Image and Weight Concerns among African American and White Adolescent Females: Differences that Make a Difference." *Human Organization* 54 (2): 103–25.

PAYNE, LUCINDA, DENISE MARTZ, BROOKE TOMPKINS NEZAMI, ANNA PETROFF, AND CLAIRE V. FARROW

2011   "Gender Comparisons of Fat Talk in the United Kingdom and the United States." *Sex Roles* 65 (7/8): 557–65.

PIESS, KATHY

1986   *Cheap Amusements: Working Women and Leisure in Turn-of-the-Century New York.* Philadelphia: Temple University Press.

2002   "Educating the Eye of the Beholder—American Cosmetics Abroad." *Daedalus* 131 (4): 101–9.

PIKE, KATHLEEN M., FAITH-ANNE DOHM, RUTH H. STRIEGEL-MOORE,
DENISE E. WILFLEY, AND CHRISTOPHER G. FAIRBURN
2001   "A Comparison of Black and White Women with Binge Eating Disorder." *American Journal of Psychiatry* 158:1455–60.

POMERANTZ, ANITA
1984   "Agreeing and Disagreeing with Assessments: Some Features of Preferred/ Dispreferred Turn Shapes." In *Structures of Social Action: Studies in Conversation Analysis*, edited by J. Maxwell Atkinson and John Heritage, 57–101. Cambridge: Cambridge University Press.

POPE, HARRISON, KATHARINE A. PHILLIPS, AND ROBERTO OLIVARDIA
2000   *The Adonis Complex: The Secret Crisis of Male Body Obsession.* New York: Simon and Shuster.

POPENOE, REBECCA
2004   *Feeding Desire: Fatness, Beauty, and Sexuality among a Saharan People.* New York: Routledge.

POPKIN, BARRY M.
2001   "The Nutrition Transition and Obesity in the Developing World." *Journal of Nutrition* 131 (3): 871S–873S.

2009   *The World Is Fat: The Fads, Trends, Policies, and Products that Are Fattening the Human Race.* New York: Penguin.

POPKIN, BARRY, LINGA ADAIR, AND SHU WEN NG
2012   "Global Nutrition Transition and the Pandemic of Obesity in Developing Countries." *Nutrition Reviews* 70 (1): 3–21.

POWELL, ANDREA D., AND ARNOLD S. KAHN
1995   "Racial Differences in Women's Desires to Be Thin." *International Journal of Eating Disorders* 17 (2): 191–95.

POWERS, RETHA
1989   "Fat Is a Black Women's Issue." *Essence* 20 (6): 75–79.

PUHL, REBECCA M., TATIANA ANDREYEVA, AND KELLY D. BROWNELL
2008   "Perceptions of Weight Discrimination: Prevalence and Comparison to Race and Gender Discrimination in America." *International Journal of Obesity* 32 (6): 992–1000.

PUHL, REBECCA, AND CHELSEA HEUER
2009   "The Stigma of Obesity: A Review and Update." *Obesity* 17:941–64.

2010   "Obesity Stigma: Important Considerations for Public Health." *American Journal of Public Health* 100 (6): 1019–28.

PUHL, REBECCA M., JANET D. LATNER, KERRY S. O'BRIEN, JOERG LUEDICKE, SIGRUN DANIELSDOTTIR, AND MARY FORHAN

2015 "A Multinational Examination of Weight Bias: Predictors of Anti-Fat Attitudes across Four Countries." *International Journal of Obesity* 1 (8): 1–8.

PUHL, REBECCA M., JAMIE LEE PETERSON, AND JOERGE LUEDICKE

2013 "Fighting Obesity or Obese Persons? Public Perceptions of Obesity-Related Health Messages." *International Journal of Obesity* 37:774–82.

PUOANE, THANDI, WITH LUNGISWA TSOLEKILE AND NELIA STEYN

2010 "Perceptions about Body Image and Sizes among Black African Girls Living in Cape Town." *Ethnicity & Disease* 20:29–34.

QUICK, VIRGINIA M., RITA MCWILLIAMS, AND CAROL BYRD-BREDBENNER

2013 "Fatty, Fatty Two-by-Four: Weight-Teasing History and Disturbed Eating in Young Adult Women." *American Journal of Public Health* 103 (3): 508–15.

RADLOFF, LENORE SAWYER

1977 "The CES-D Scale a Self-Report Depression Scale for Research in the General Population." *Applied Psychological Measurement* 1 (3): 385–401.

RASMUSSEN, KATHLEEN M., AND ANN L. YAKTINE, EDS.

2009 *Weight Gain during Pregnancy: Reexamining the Guidelines.* Washington, DC: National Academies Press.

RASMUSSEN, SUSAN J.

2010a "Debating Beauties (a Three-Way Comparison of Bodily Aesthetics)." In *Tuareg Society within a Globalized World: Saharan Life in Transition*, edited by Anja Fischer and Ines Kohl, 125–43. London: I. B. Tauris Press.

2010b "Remaking Body Politics: Dilemmas over Female Fatness as Symbolic Capital in Two Rural Tuareg Communities." *Culture, Medicine, and Psychiatry* 34 (4): 615–32.

RAVUVU, ASESELA

1983 *Vaka i Taukei: The Fijian Way of Life.* Suva, Fiji: Institute of Pacific Studies of the University of the South Pacific.

REISCHER, ERICA, AND KATHRYN S. KOO

2004 "The Body Beautiful: Symbolism and Agency in the Social World." *Annual Review of Anthropology* 33:297–317.

REYNOLDS WHYTE, SUSAN

2014 "The Publics of the New Public Health: Life Conditions and 'Lifestyle Diseases' in Uganda." In *Making and Unmaking Public Health in Africa: Ethnographic and Historical Perspectives*, edited by Ruth J. Prince and Rebecca Marsland. Athens: Ohio University Press.

RICHIE, BETH E.

2012   *Arrested Justice: Black Women, Violence, and America's Prison Nation.* New
        York: New York University Press.

RITENBAUGH, CHERYL

1982   "Obesity as a Culture-Bound Syndrome." *Culture, Medicine, and Psychiatry*
        6 (4): 347–61.

ROBERTO, CHRISTINE, BOYD SWINBURN, CORINNA HAWKES, TERRY T.-K. HUANG,
SERGIO A. COSTA, MARICE ASHE, LINDSEY ZWICKER, JOHN H. CAWLEY, AND
KELLY D. BROWNELL

2015   "Patchy Progress on Obesity Prevention: Emerging Examples, Entrenched
        Barriers, and New Thinking." *Lancet* 385 (9985): 2400–2409.

ROBERTS, ANDREW, JENNIFER KING, AND FRANK GREENWAY

2004   "Class III Obesity Continues to Rise in African-American Women." *Obesity
        Surgery* 14 (4): 533–35.

ROBERTS, DOROTHY

1997   *Killing the Black Body: Race, Reproduction, and the Meaning of Liberty.* New
        York: Pantheon Books.

ROGGE, MARY M.

2004   "Obesity, Stigma, and Civilized Oppression." *Advances in Nursing Science*
        27 (4): 301–15.

ROHDE, DAVID

2011   "Free-Falling in Milwaukee: A Close-Up on One City's Middle-Class
        Decline." *Atlantic*, December 16.

ROSSITER, ELISE M., AND W. STEWART AGRAS

1990   "An Empirical Test of the DSM-III-R Definition of Binge." *International
        Journal of Eating Disorders* 9 (5): 513–18.

ROTHBLUM, ESTHER

1992   "The Stigma of Women's Weight: Social and Economic Realities." *Feminism
        & Psychology* 2:61–73.

ROTHBLUM, ESTHER, AND SONDRA SOLOVAY, EDS.

2009   *The Fat Studies Reader.* New York: New York University Press.

RUBIN LISA R., MAKO L. FITTS, AND ANNE E. BECKER

2003   "'Whatever Feels Good in My Soul': Body Ethics and Aesthetics among Afri-
        can American and Latina Women." *Culture, Medicine, and Psychiatry* 27 (1):
        49–75.

RUIZ, REBECCA

2007   "In Pictures: America's Most Obese Cities." *Forbes*, November 14. http://
        www.forbes.com/2007/11/14/health-obesity-cities-forbeslife-cx_rr_1114bese
        _slide_10.html.

RUSH, E. C., I. FREITAS, AND L. D. PLANK

2009   "Body Size, Body Composition and Fat Distribution: Comparative Analysis of European, Maori, Pacific Island and Asian Indian Adults." *British Journal of Nutrition* 102:632–41.

RYAN, TRAVIS A., TODD G. MORRISON, AND CORMAC Ó BEAGLAOICH

2010   "Adolescent Males' Body Image: An Overview of Research on the Influence of Mass Media." In *Boys' Bodies: Speaking the Unspoken*, edited by Michael Kehler and Michael Atkinson, 153–75. New York: Peter Lang.

SABIK, NATALIE J., ELIZABETH R. COLE, AND L. MONIQUE WARD

2010   "Are All Minority Women Equally Buffered from Negative Body Image? Intra-Ethnic Moderators of the Buffering Hypothesis." *Psychology of Women Quarterly* 34 (2): 139–51.

SAGUY, ABIGAIL C.

2013   *What's Wrong with Fat?* New York: Oxford University Press.

SAGUY, ABIGAIL C., AND KJERSTIN GRUYS

2010   "Morality and Health: News Media Constructions of Overweight and Eating Disorders." *Social Problems* 57 (2): 231–50.

SAGUY, ABIGAIL C., KJERSTIN GRUYS, AND SHANNA GONG

2010   "Social Problem Construction and National Context: News Reporting on 'Overweight' and 'Obesity' in the US and France." *Social Problems* 57 (4): 586–610.

SAINZ, ADRIAN

2013   "Memphis Makes Progress in Infant Mortality Fight." Associated Press, March 1.

SALIHU, HAMISU M., AMINA P. ALIO, RONÉE E. WILSON, PUZA P. SHARMA, RUSSELL S. KIRBY, AND GREG R. ALEXANDER

2008   "Obesity and Extreme Obesity: New Insights into the Black-White Disparity in Neonatal Mortality." *Obstetrics and Gynecology* 111 (6): 1410–16.

SALK, RACHEL, AND RENEE ENGELN-MADDOX

2012   "Fat Talk among College Women Is both Contagious and Harmful." *Sex Roles* 66 (9/10): 636–45.

SANDERS, TEELA, AND KATE HARDY

2012   "Devalued, Deskilled and Diversified: Explaining the Proliferation of the Strip Industry in the UK." *British Journal of Sociology* 63:513–32.

SANDERS-PHILLIPS, KATHY, BEVERLYN SETTLES-REAVES, DOREN WALKER, AND JANEESE BROWNLOW

2009   "Social Inequality and Racial Discrimination: Risk Factors for Health Disparities in Children of Color." *Pediatrics* 124:S176.

SAUVAKACOLO, SITERI

2014   "Substance Abuse." *Fiji Times*, February 19. http://www.fijitimes.com/story
        .aspx?id=260358. Accessed March 6, 2015.

SCARRY, ELAINE

2001   *On Beauty and Being Just*. Princeton, NJ: Princeton University Press.

SCHEPER-HUGHES, NANCY, AND MARGARET M. LOCK

1987   "The Mindful Body: A Prolegomenon to Future Work in Medical Anthro-
        pology." *Medical Anthropology Quarterly* 1 (1): 6–41.

SCHLAERTH, KATHERINE

2014   "Science Doesn't Lie—Modern Mothers Are Lazier." *SFGate.com*,
        January 20. http://www.sfgate.com/opinion/openforum/article/Science-
        doesn-t-lie-modern-mothers-are-lazier-5160269.php.

SCHULZ, AMY J., AND LEITH MULLINGS, EDS.

2006   *Gender, Race, Class and Health: Intersectional Approaches*. Hoboken, NJ:
        Wiley and Sons.

SCHWARTZ, HILLEL

1986   *Never Satisfied: A Cultural History of Diets, Fantasies, and Fat*. New York:
        Free Press.

SCHWARTZ, MARLENE B., AND KELLY D. BROWNELL

2007   "Actions Necessary to Prevent Childhood Obesity: Creating the Climate for
        Change." *Journal of Law, Medicine, & Ethics* 35 (1): 78–89.

SHAIKH, H., S. ROBINSON, AND T. G. TEOH

2010   "Management of Maternal Obesity Prior to and during Pregnancy." *Seminars
        in Fetal and Neonatal Medicine* 15:77–82.

SHARPE, HELEN, ULRIKE NAUMAN, JANET TREASURE, AND ULRIKE SCHMIDT

2013   "Is Fat Talking a Causal Risk Factor for Body Dissatisfaction? A Systematic
        Review and Meta-Analysis." *International Journal of Eating Disorders* 46:
        643–52.

SHILDRICK, MARGRIT, AND JANET PRICE

1998   *Vital Signs: Feminist Reconfigurations of the Bio/logical Body*. Edinburgh:
        Edinburgh University Press.

SHILLING, CHRIS

1993   *The Body and Social Theory*. London: Sage.

SHIM, JANET K.

2002   "Understanding the Routinized Inclusion of Race, Socioeconomic Status and
        Sex in Epidemiology: The Utility of Concepts from Technoscience Studies."
        Sociology of Health and Illness 24:129–50.

2014   *Heart Sick: The Politics of Risk, Inequality, and Heart Disease*. New York: New
        York University Press.

SILVERSTEIN, BRETT, LAUREN PERDUE, BARBARA PETERSON, LINDA VOGEL, AND
DEBORAH A. FANTINI
1986   "Possible Causes of the Thin Standard of Bodily Attractiveness for Women."
        International Journal of Eating Disorders 5 (5): 907–16.

SIMMONS, WILLIAM PAUL, AND MONICA J. CASPER
2012   "Culpability, Social Triage, and Structural Violence in the Aftermath of
        Katrina." *Perspectives on Politics* 10 (3): 675–86.

SIMPSON, S. J., AND D. RAUBENHEIMER
2005   "Obesity: The Protein Leverage Hypothesis." *Obesity Reviews* 6:133–42.

SINGH, DEVENDRA
1993   "Adaptive Significance of Female Physical Attractiveness: Role of Waist-to-
        Hip Ratio." *Journal of Personality and Social Psychology* 65 (2): 293–307.

SKOCPOL, THEDA
1992   *Protecting Soldiers and Mothers: The Political Origins of Social Policy in the
        United States.* Cambridge: Harvard University Press.

SMITH, DARRON T.
2013   "The Epigenetics of Being Black and Feeling Blue: Understanding African
        American Vulnerability to Disease." *HuffingtonPost.com*, October 14. http://
        www.huffingtonpost.com/darron-t-smith-phd/the-epigenetics-of-being
        -_b_4094226.html.

SMITH, DELIA E., J. KEVIN THOMPSON, JAMES M. RACZYNSKI, AND JOAN E. HILNER
1999   "Body Image among Men and Women in a Biracial Cohort: The CARDIA
        Study." *International Journal of Eating Disorders* 25 (1): 71–82.

SOBAL, JEFFERY
1991   "Obesity and Nutritional Sociology: A Model for Coping with the Stigma of
        Obesity." *Clinical Sociology Review* 9 (1): 125–41.

1995   "The Medicalization and Demedicalization of Obesity." In *Eating Agendas:
        Food and Nutrition as Social Problems*, edited by Donna Maurer and Jeffery
        Sobal, 67–90. New York: Walter de Gruyter.

SOBAL, J., AND A. J. STUNKARD
1989   "Socioeconomic Status and Obesity: A Review of the Literature." *Psychologi-
        cal Bulletin* 105 (2): 260–75.

SOBH, RANA, RUSSELL BELK, AND JUSTIN GRESSEL
2014   "Mimicry and Modernity in the Middle East: Fashion Invisibility and Young
        Women of the Arab Gulf." *Consumption Markets and Culture* 17 (4): 392–412.

SOBO, ELIZA
1993   *One Blood: The Jamaican Body.* Albany: State University of New York Press.

1994   "The Sweetness of Fat: Health, Procreation, and Sociability in Rural Jamaica."

In *Many Mirrors: Body Image and Social Meaning*, edited by Nicole Sault, 132–54. New Brunswick, NJ: Rutgers University Press.

STAFFORD, MARK C., AND RICHARD R. SCOTT

1986   "Stigma, Deviance, and Social Control." In *The Dilemma of Difference: A Multidisciplinary View of Stigma*, edited by S. C. Ainlay, G. Becker, and L. M. Coleman, 77–91. New York: Springer.

STEARNS, PETER

2002   *Fat History: Bodies and Beauty in the Modern West*. New York: New York University Press.

STEINER-ADAIR, CATHERINE

1978   "Weightism: A New Form of Prejudice." *National Anorexic Aid Society Newsletter* 10(4).

STERN, MARILYN, SUZANNE E. MAZZEO, JERLYM PORTER, CLARICE GERKE, DAPHNE BRYAN, AND JOSEPH LAVER

2006   "Self-Esteem, Teasing and Quality of Life: African American Adolescent Girls Participating in a Family-Based Pediatric Overweight Intervention." *Journal of Clinical Psychology in Medical Settings* 13 (3): 217–28.

STORMER, NATHAN

2000   "Prenatal Space." *Signs* 26 (1): 109–44.

STRAUSS, ANSELM

1978   *Negotiations: Varieties, Processes, Contexts, and Social Order*. San Francisco: Jossey-Bass.

STRAUSS, RICHARD, AND HAROLD POLLACK

2003   "Social Marginalization of Overweight Children." *Archives of Pediatrics & Adolescent Medicine* 157:746–52.

STRIEGEL-MOORE, RUTH H., AND CYNTHIA M. BULIK

2007   "Risk Factors for Eating Disorders." *American Psychologist* 62 (3): 181–98.

SUBRAMANIAN, S. V., JESSICA M. PERKINS, EMRE ÖZALTIN, AND GEORGE DAVEY SMITH

2011   "Weight of Nations: A Socioeconomic Analysis of Women in Low- to Middle-Income Countries." *American Journal of Clinical Nutrition* 93:413–21.

SUNDBORN, GERHARD, WITH PATRICIA A. METCALF, DUDLEY GENTLES, ROBERT K. SCRAGG, DAVID SCHAAF, LORNA DYALL, PETER BLACK, AND ROD JACKSON

2008   "Ethnic Differences in Cardiovascular Disease Risk Factors and Diabetes Status for Pacific Ethnic Groups and Europeans in the Diabetes Heart and Health Survey (DHAH) 2002–2003, Auckland New Zealand." *New Zealand Medical Journal* 121 (1281): 28–39.

SWEET, ELIZABETH

2011   "Symbolic Capital, Consumption, and Health Inequality." *American Journal of Public Health* 101:260–64.

TALLEY, HEATHER LAINE

2014   *Saving Face: Disfigurement and the Politics of Appearance.* New York: New York University Press.

TALUKDAR, JAITA

2012   "Thin but Not Skinny: Women Negotiating the 'Never Too Thin' Body Ideal in Urban India." *Women's Studies International Forum* 35:109–18.

TAYLOR, NICOLE

2006   "Constructing Gendered Identities through Discourse: Body Image, Exercise, Food Consumption, and Teasing Practices among Adolescents." PhD diss., University of Arizona.

2011a   "'Guys, She's Humongous!': Gender and Weight-Based Teasing in Adolescence." *Journal of Adolescent Research* 26 (2): 178–99.

2011b   "Negotiating Popular Obesity Discourses in Adolescence: School Food, Personal Responsibility, and Gendered Food Consumption Behaviors." *Food, Culture, & Society* 14 (4): 587–606.

2016   *Schooled on Fat: What Teens Tell Us about Gender, Body Image, and Obesity.* New York: Routledge.

TENNANT, P. W. G., J. RANKIN, AND R. BELL

2011   "Maternal Body Mass Index and the Risk of Fetal and Infant Death: A Cohort Study from the North of England." *Human Reproduction* 26 (6): 1501–11.

THOMAS, DUNCAN, AND JOHN STRAUSS

1997   "Health and Wages: Evidence on Men and Women in Urban Brazil." *Journal of Econometrics* 77 (1): 159–85.

THOMAS, JENNIFER J., ROSS D. CROSBY, STEPHEN A. WONDERLICH, RUTH H. STRIEGEL-MOORE, AND ANNE E. BECKER

2011   "A Latent Profile Analysis of the Typology of Bulimic Symptoms in an Indigenous Pacific Population: Evidence of Cross-Cultural Variation in Phenomenology." *Psychological Medicine* 41 (1): 195–206.

THOMAS, JENNIFER J., AND JENNI SCHAEFER

2013   *Almost Anorexic: Is My (or My Loved One's) Relationship with Food a Problem?* Center City, MN: Hazelden.

THOMAS, MARTINA

2010   "Perceptions of Body Image among Low Socioeconomic Status African American Mothers and Their Daughters in Mobile, Alabama." Master's thesis, University of Alabama.

THOMAS, SAMANTHA L., JIM HYDE, ASUNTHA KARUNARATNE, DILINIE HERBERT, AND
PAUL A. KOMESAROFF

2008   "Being 'Fat' in Today's World: A Qualitative Study of the Lived Experiences
        of People with Obesity in Australia." *Health Expectations* 11 (4): 321–30.

THOMPSON, BECKY W.

1994   *A Hunger So Wide and So Deep: American Women Speak Out on Eating Prob-*
        lems. Minneapolis: University of Minnesota Press.

THOMPSON, DANIEL R., CHERYL L. CLARK, BETSY WOOD, AND MARY BETH ZENI

2008   "Maternal Obesity and Risk of Infant Death Based on Florida Birth Records
        for 2004." *Public Health Reports* 123 (4): 487–93.

TOMISAKA, KAZUE, JIMAIMA LAKO, CHIZUKO MARUYAMA, NGUYEN THI LAN ANH,
DO THI KIM LIEN, HA HUY KHOI, AND NGUYEN VAN CHUYEN

2002   "Dietary Patterns and Risk Factors for Type 2 Diabetes Mellitus in Fijian,
        Japanese and Vietnamese Populations." *Asia Pacific Journal of Clinical Nutri-*
        tion 11 (1): 8–12.

TORLONI, MARIA REGINA, ANA PILAR BERTRAN, AND MARIO MERIALDI

2012   "Demography of Obesity." In *Maternal Obesity*, edited by Matthew W. Gill-
        man and Lucilla Poston, 1–7. Cambridge: Cambridge University Press.

TRAINER, SARAH

2012   "Negotiating Weight and Body Image in the UAE: Strategies among Young
        Emirati Women." *American Journal of Human Biology* 24:314–24. Special
        Issue on Global Obesity.

2013a   "Body Image and Weight Concerns among Emirati Women in the United
        Arab Emirates." In *Reconstructing Obesity: The Measure of Meaning, the*
        Meaning of Measures, edited by J. Hardin and M. McCullough. New York:
        Berghahn Books.

2013b   "Local Interpretations of Global Trends: Body Concerns and Self-Projects
        Enacted by Young Emirati Women." PhD diss., University of Arizona.

TRAINER, SARAH, ALEXANDRA BREWIS, DEBORAH WILLIAMS, AND JOSE CHAVEZ

2015a   "Obese, Fat, or 'Just Big'? Young Adult Deployment of and Reactions to
        Weight Terms." *Human Organization* 74 (3): 266–75.

TRAINER, SARAH, DANIEL HRUSCHKA, DEBORAH WILLIAMS, AND ALEXANDRA BREWIS

2015b   "Translating Obesity: Navigating the Front Lines of the 'War on Fat.'" *Ameri-*
        can Journal of Human Biology 27 (1): 61–68.

TRAUTNER, MARY NEIL

2005   "Doing Gender, Doing Class: The Performance of Sexuality in Exotic Dance
        Clubs." *Gender & Society* 19:771–88.

TURNER, BRYAN S.

1982   "The Discourse of Diet." *Theory, Culture & Society* 1 (1): 23–32.

1984   *The Body and Society: Explorations in Social Theory*. Oxford: Basil Blackwell.

ULIJASZEK, STANLEY J.

2001   "Increasing Body Size among Adult Cook Islanders between 1966 and 1996."
        Annals of Human Biology 28 (4): 363–73.

UNITED ARAB EMIRATES (UAE)

2014   *Official Portal of the UAE*. http://government.ae/en/web/guest/open-data.
        Accessed May 1, 2014.

UNITED ARAB EMIRATES MINISTRY OF EDUCATION (UAE MINISTRY OF EDUCATION)

2014   *Education in the UAE*. https://www.moe.gov.ae/English/Pages/UAE/UaeEdu
        .aspx. Accessed May 1, 2014.

UNITED ARAB EMIRATES MINISTRY OF STATE FOR FEDERAL NATIONAL COUNCIL
AFFAIRS (UAE MINISTRY OF STATE)

2008   *Women in the UAE: A Portrait of Progress*. Abu Dhabi: United Arab Emirates.

UNITED NATIONS AND LEAGUE OF ARAB STATES (UN AND LEAGUE)

2013   *The Arab Millennium Development Goals Report: Facing Challenges and
        Looking Beyond 2015*. UNDP Report. Beirut: ESCWA.

US BUREAU OF THE CENSUS

2012   American Fact Finder. Five-year estimates, 2006–2010. http://factfinder2
        .census.gov/faces/nav/jsf/pages/index.xhtml. Accessed October 16, 2012.

VANNUCCI, ANNA, KELLY R. THEIM, ANDREA E. KASS, MICKEY TROCKEL, BROOKE
GENKIN, MARIANNE RIZK, HANNAH WEISMAN, J. O. BAILEY, M. M. SINTON, V. ASPEN,
D. E. WILFLEY, AND C. B. TAYLOR

2013   "What Constitutes Clinically Significant Binge Eating? Association between
        Binge Features and Clinical Validators in College-Age Women." *Interna-
        tional Journal of Eating Disorders* 46 (3): 226–32.

VINAYAGAM, DIMUTHU, AND EDWIN CHANDRAHARAN

2012   "The Adverse Impact of Maternal Obesity on Intrapartum and Perinatal
        Outcomes." *ISRN Obstetrics and Gynecology*. http://www.hindawi.com/isrn
        /obgyn/2012/939762.

WACQUANT, LOIC

1995   "Pugs at Work: Bodily Capital and Bodily Labour among Professional Box-
        ers." *Body & Society* 1:65–93.

WADA, ROY, AND ERDAL TEKIN

2010   "Body Composition and Wages." *Economics & Human Biology* 8 (2): 242–54.

WALD, ELIJAH

2012   *The Dozens: A History of Rap's Mama*. New York: Oxford University Press.

WALKER, RENEE E., CHRISTOPHER R. KEANE, AND JESSICA G. BURKE
2010   "Disparities and Access to Healthy Food in the United States: A Review of Food Deserts Literature." *Health and Place* 16 (5): 876–84.

WALLER, WILLARD
1937   "The Rating and Dating Complex." *American Sociological Review* 2 (5): 727–34.

WARHURST, CHRIS, AND DENNIS NICKSON
2009   "'Who's Got the Look?' Emotional, Aesthetic and Sexualized Labour in Interactive Services." *Gender, Work and Organization* 16:385–404.

WEBB, TAMMY T., E. JOAN LOOBY, AND REGINA FULTS-MCMURTERY
2004   "African American Men's Perceptions of Body Figure Attractiveness: An Acculturation Study." *Journal of Black Studies* 34 (3): 370–85.

WEBSTER, MURRAY, AND JAMES DRISKELL
1983   "Beauty as Status." *American Journal of Sociology* 89: 140–65.

WELLS, J. C. K.
2009   *The Evolutionary Biology of Human Body Fatness.* Cambridge: Cambridge University Press.

WILK, RICHARD
1995   "Learning to Be Local in Belize: Global Systems of Common Difference." In *Worlds Apart: Modernity through the Prism of the Local*, edited by Daniel Miller, 110–33. London: Routledge.

WILLIAMS, CHRISTINE L., AND CATHERINE CONNELL
2010   "'Looking Good and Sounding Right': Aesthetic Labor and Social Inequality in the Retail Industry." *Work and Occupations* 37:349–77.

WILLIAMS, DAVID
2005   "Social Sources of Racial Disparities in Health." *Health Affairs* 24 (2): 325–34.

WOLF, NAOMI
1990   *The Beauty Myth: How Images of Beauty Are Used against Women.* 1st ed. New York: Vintage.

1991   *The Beauty Myth: How Images of Beauty Are Used against Women.* 2nd ed. New York: Harper.

WOLFE, BARBARA E., CHRISTINA W. BAKER, ADRIAN T. SMITH, AND SUSAN KELLY-WEEDER
2009   "Validity and Utility of the Current Definition of Binge Eating." *International Journal of Eating Disorders* 42 (8): 674–86.

WORLD HEALTH ORGANIZATION (WHO)
2004   *Obesity: Preventing and Managing the Global Epidemic.* Report of a WHO Consultation. Geneva: WHO.

2014a   "BMI Classification." World Health Organization, http://apps.who.int/bmi
        /index.jsp?introPage=intro_3.html. Accessed September 2014.

2014b   "Chronic Diseases and Health Promotion." World Health Organization,
        http://www.who.int/chp/en/index.html. Accessed September 2014.

2014c   "Overweight/Obesity: Overweight (Body Mass Index > 25): Data by Coun-
        try." World Health Organization, http://apps.who.int/gho/data/node.main
        .A897. Accessed September 2014.

2014d   "Overweight/Obesity: Obesity (Body Mass Index > 30): Data by Country."
        World Health Organization, http://apps.who.int/gho/data/node.main.A900
        ?lang=en. Accessed September 2014.

2014e   "Preventing Chronic Diseases: A Vital Investment." World Health Organiza-
        tion, http://www.who.int/chp/chronic_disease_report/en. Accessed Septem-
        ber 2014.

2014f   "The Impact of Chronic Disease in the United Arab Emirates." World Health
        Organization, http://www.who.int/chp/chronic_disease_report/uae.pdf.
        Accessed September 2014.

2015a   "Controlling the Global Obesity Epidemic." WHO Fact Sheet. World Health
        Organization, http://www.who.int/nutrition/topics/obesity/en. Accessed
        June 1, 2015.

2015b   "Media Center: Obesity and Overweight." WHO Fact Sheet. World Health
        Organization, http://www.who.int/mediacentre/factsheets/fs311/en. Accessed
        January 15, 2015.

2015c   "Prevalence of Overweight, Ages 18+, 2010–2014 (Age Standardized Esti-
        mate)." World Health Organization, http://www.who.int/healthinfo/indica
        tors/2015/chi_2015_67_adults_overweight.pdf?ua=1. Accessed June 1, 2015.

WORLD HEALTH ORGANIZATION, EASTERN MEDITERRANEAN REGION (WHO-EMRO)
2003   "WHO Global Strategy on Diet, Physical Activity and Health." In *Eastern
        Mediterranean Regional Consultation Meeting Report*. Cairo: WHO.

2014a   "Noncommunicable Diseases." World Health Organization, http://www
        .emro.who.int/ncd. Accessed September 2014.

2014b   "United Arab Emirates." World Health Organization, http://www.who.int
        /nmh/countries/are_en.pdf. Accessed September 2014.

YACH, DEREK, DAVID STUCKLER, AND KELLY D. BROWNELL
2006   "Corrigendum: Epidemiologic and Economic Consequences of the Global
        Epidemics of Obesity and Diabetes." *Nature Medicine* 12 (3): 62–66.

YANCEY, ANTRONETTE K., JOANNE LESLIE, AND EMILY K. ABEL
2006   "Obesity at the Crossroads: Feminist and Public Health Perspectives." *Signs*
        31 (2): 425–43.

YANG, LAWRENCE H., FANG-PEI CHEN, KATHLEEN JANEL SIA, JONATHAN LAM,
KATHERINE LAM, HONG NGO, SING LEE, ARTHUR KLEINMAN, AND BYRON GOODE
2014   "What Matters Most: A Cultural Mechanism Moderating Structural Vulnera-
          bility and Moral Experience of Mental Illness Stigma." *Social Science and
          Medicine* 103:84–93.

YOUNG, IRIS MARION
2005   *On Female Body Experience: "Throwing Like a Girl" and Other Essays.* New
          York: Oxford University Press.

ZHANG, QI, AND YOUFA WANG
2004   "Socioeconomic Inequality of Obesity in the United States: Do Gender, Age,
          and Ethnicity Matter?" *Social Science and Medicine* 58 (6): 1171–80.

ZUCKERMAN, DIANA
2010   "Reasonably Safe? Breast Implants and Informed Consent." *Reproductive
          Health Matters* 18 (35): 94–102.

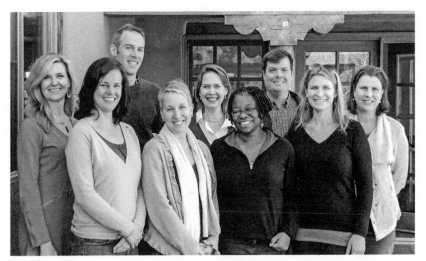

Participants in the School for Advanced Research advanced seminar "Obesity, Upward Mobility, and Symbolic Body Capital in a Rapidly Changing World," co-chaired by Eileen Anderson-Fye and Alexandra Brewis, March 2–6, 2014. *Standing in back row, from left*: Alexander Edmonds, Anne E. Becker, Daniel J. Hruschka, and Alexandra Brewis. *Standing in front row, from left*: Eileen Anderson-Fye, Nicole L. Taylor, Monica J. Casper, Stephanie M. McClure, and Sarah Trainer. Photograph by Cynthia Geoghegan.

EILEEN P. ANDERSON-FYE
Department of Bioethics, Case Western Reserve University

ANNE E. BECKER, MD, PHD, MPH
Department of Global Health and Social Medicine, Harvard Medical School

ARUNDHATI BHARATI
Department of Anthropology, Case Western Reserve University

ALEXANDRA BREWIS
School of Human Evolution and Social Change, Arizona State University

MONICA J. CASPER
College of Social and Behavioral Sciences, University of Arizona

YUNZHU CHEN
Department of Anthropology, Case Western Reserve University

ALEXANDER EDMONDS
Department of Social Anthropology, University of Edinburgh

MAUREEN FLORIANO
Department of Anthropology, Case Western Reserve University

DANIEL J. HRUSCHKA
Department of Anthropology, School for Human Evolution and Social Change, Arizona State University

CARYL JAMES
Department of Sociology, Psychology and Social Work, University of the West Indies

REBECCA J. LESTER
Department of Anthropology, Washington University in St. Louis

STEPHANIE M. MCCLURE
Department of Behavioral Science and Health Education, Saint Louis
   University

ASHLEY MEARS
Department of Sociology, Boston University

NICOLE L. TAYLOR
Department of Anthropology, Texas State University

SARAH TRAINER
 School for Human Evolution and Social Change, Arizona State University

Index

and, 67–69; labor fields and, 38; with
weight management techniques, 42,
44–47; WHR, 106
body-size ideals: body image and, 101–5;
obesity stigma with instrumentality,
gender, and, 57–59; race and, 98–99
body-wealth associations: body mass
reversal and, 19–23; females and,
15; food and, 16; males and, 15; with
obesity, BMI, and SES, 17–19, 29, 200;
reversal of, 8–9, 15–16
body weight: BMI with height and, 88;
family with management of, 151–52, 166,
202–3; Fiji with diet, social health, and,
152–54; friends and negotiating, 185–87;
men, romance, and, 187–91; with shape,
management techniques, 42, 44–47;
social mobility with social change and,
159–60. *See also* United Arab Emirates,
body weight and image in
Bollywood movies, 73, 75, 182
Bordo, Susan, 126, 198
Bourdieu, Pierre, 7, 33, 36, 37, 38
boys: with gendered identities, "pulling
off," 132–36; with romance and body
weight, 187–91; verbal dueling among,
142–46. *See also* language, youth with
body and
brain, neuro-circuitry, 157
Brazil: plastic surgery in, 33, 39–40, 46;
"sofa audition" in, 41
Brewis, Alexandra A., 127
Bucholtz, Mary, 129
bulimia nervosa, 156, 167
Butler, Judith, 125, 146

Canada, 164
capital, 33, 36. *See also* body capital; contingent capital; erotic capital; sexual
capital; social capital; symbolic capital
care, in Fiji: defined, 153; with overeating
and social values, 154–55

caste, social hierarchy, 78n2
censure, body capital, attractiveness, and,
105–8
character judgments, in Nepal, 72
chiefly governance, tradition with, 159
children, soldiering and, 78n1. *See also*
boys; girls
China: beauty in, 35, 42; obesity in, 2; sex
work in, 42, 48n1; wealth and BMI in,
27
class, with gender and race, 110–11. *See
also* social hierarchy
Coca-Cola shape, 61, 67, 112, 128
Collins, James, Jr., 87
color, attractiveness and, 40
competition. *See* cooperative competition, among girls
contingent capital: in context, 111; "curvy"
and well dressed, 118–21, *119*; dating
and being too skinny, 115–18, *116*; "fat,
not curvy," 112–15, *113*
control: of body, 111, 125; loss of, 157. *See
also* eating disorders
cooperative competition, among girls,
139–42, 198
costs, of obesity, 49
culture: beauty standards and, 34–35, 42;
body image with cultural protection,
101–2; embodied cultural capital, 33,
36; multiple body ideals, 61–62; racialized bodies within, 100–101, 107–8
"curvy": not fat, 112–15, *113*; well dressed
and, 118–21, *119*

dating: with being too skinny, 115–18, *116*;
body capital and, 106; online, 42
David, Richard, 87
depression, 50, 164–65, 194
*Diagnostic and Statistical Manual of Men-
tal Disorders* (DSM-IV), 152, 155
diet, in Fiji, 152–54
disciplinary power, 129–30, 138

disparagement, of fat, 57, 100–101, 108, 134–35, 150
dissatisfaction, with body, 97, 102, 123n2, 178, 201
distribution, of fat, 69
dress: abaya as national, 172, 177, 179, 188, 190; shayla as national, 172, 177. *See also* well dressed
DSM-IV. *See Diagnostic and Statistical Manual of Mental Disorders*
Du Bois, W. E. B., 97, 122, 194

eating disorders, 44, 194; anorexia nervosa, 46, 76, 157, 165, 203; BED, 155–56, 158; bulimia nervosa, 156, 167; globalization of, 151–52; modeling and, 45; parents influencing, 151–52, 202–3; triggers, 157. *See also* obesity; overeating, in Fiji
Eckert, Penelope, 141–42
economic model, limitations of, 202–3
economy: with height influencing salaries, 36; obesity, cost of, 49; prosperity and "tipping point" in, 49–50; with salaries and gender, 30; SES, 17–19, 29, 200; sex work, 42, 48n1. *See also* labor fields
Eder, Donna, 143
Edmonds, Alexander, 39, 40, 196–97
Egypt, 18–19
Eisenstein, Zillah, 83
"elective sexuality," 41
embodied cultural capital, 33, 36
employment, with upward mobility, 61. *See also* labor fields
epidemic, obesity as, 79–80, 125–26, 173
erotic capital: attributes of, 48n1; gender inequality and, 34, 37–38
Eurasia, 20, *21*, 31
Evans, Catherine Colleen, 143
exceptions, experience of being, 97, 101–5

family: body projects negotiated with,

184–85; management of body weight by, 151–52, 166, 202–3; parental occupations, *160*. *See also* boys; girls; language, youth with body and
fat: belly rolls, 56, 197; body capital and, 47–48, 100, 106–7; connotations, 52, 56, 62–63, 72, 90, 127, 175, 179; disparagement, 57, 100–101, 108, 134–35, 150; distribution, 69; laziness and, 127, 129; mass, 17, 18, 27; meanings of, 193–95; modernization and, 179–80; not curvy, 112–15, *113*; positive attitudes about, 2, 175; shaming, 47, 89; value of, 34, 47–48, 100, 194. *See also* obesity
fat-free mass. *See* lean mass
fat stigma, 4, 50; global spread of, 2–3, 10, 49, 128; prevalence of, 3, 137–38, 150; risk and protective factors for, 59–77; symbolic capital model and, 5–6, 7. *See also* obesity stigma
fat talk, 140–42, 150, 187
female gaze, opposite-sex attraction and, 143–44
females: beauty and tradition, 174–85, 190; with body-wealth associations, reversal of, 15; gender with size and opposite-sex attraction, 69–70; with wealth and BMI increase, 20, 22. *See also* African American females, body capital of
fetal surgery, 82
Fiji: body-ideal changes, history of, 151–52; with body ideals decoded, 167–68; with care, defined, 153; in context, 11–12, 149–50, 169, 197, 202; diet, body weight, and social health in, 152–54; diet and health in, 154; overeating and stigma in, 157–58; parental and aspirational occupations, *160*; social change and mobility with body weight in, 159–60; social construction of overeating in, 155–56; social values, care, and "overeating" in, 154–55; television,